Distal Radius Fractures

Jeffrey N. Lawton
Editor and Author

Distal Radius Fractures

A Clinical Casebook

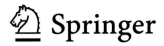 Springer

Editor and Author
Jeffrey N. Lawton
Department of Orthopedic Surgery
University of Michigan Health System
A. Alfred Taubman Health Care Center
Ann Arbor, MI, USA

ISBN 978-3-319-27487-4   ISBN 978-3-319-27489-8   (eBook)
DOI 10.1007/978-3-319-27489-8

Library of Congress Control Number: 2016935863

Printed on acid-free paper

This Springer imprint is published by Springer Nature
The registered company is Springer International Publishing AG Switzerland

Preface

I am especially proud of this assembled work *Distal Radius Fractures: A Clinical Casebook*. Along with my notable coauthors, we were able to micro-dissect the clinical care of distal radius fractures and go far beyond what is commonly seen in their presentations and other textbooks. The inspiration for this work was based upon a number of Instructional Course Lectures and the now increasingly tired mantra that I use with our Residents and Fellows in Hand Surgery that in order to take care of patients with distal radius fractures, one must be facile with a number of different treatment alternatives.

In decades gone by, surgeons could treat distal radius fractures with a dorsal plate or with an external fixator and feel that that was the appropriate way to address distal radius fractures and that could be their one or two go-to methods of treatment. However, with the explosion of different modalities to treat distal radius fractures—most notably including the volar locking plate, there has been a trend toward treatment of all distal radius fractures with a single "one size fits all" method of treatment. Unfortunately, this has resulted in insufficient or inappropriate treatment of a number of patients with distal radius fractures. The goal of this clinical compendium is to highlight a number of different facets of treatment of distal radius fractures with chapters each designed around a clinical case to demonstrate a different component of a distal radius fracture, reviewing the literature, and then getting back to that clinical case and how it was treated and then, as appropriate, to review some clinical pearls. Toward the end of the book, a specific review of some common complications is seen associated with distal radius fractures that were reviewed as well.

I am quite proud of the work we have assembled representing some of the finest centers and the thought-leaders of hand care throughout America. I believe the team of authors that this represents has made a substantial contribution to the clinical care of distal radius fractures, and I appreciate the significant amount of work that all of my colleagues have put into this collected effort. I would also like to acknowledge the work of my editors, Kristopher Spring and Brian Halm at Springer, USA, for helping me to put this collection together. Finally, I would like to acknowledge Nancy Phillips, my administrative assistant at the University of Michigan, who has helped me to organize, transcribe, collate, complete, and just generally produce this fine work that you see before you.

Ann Arbor, MI, USA   Jeffrey N. Lawton

Contents

Contributors

Jamie Cowan, MD Department of Orthopaedic Surgery, University of Michigan Health System, A. Alfred Taubman Health Care Center, Ann Arbor, MI, USA

Michael Darowish, MD Department of Orthopaedic Surgery, Penn State Milton S. Hershey Medical Center, Hershey, PA, USA

David G. Dennison, MD Department of Orthopedic Surgery, Mayo Clinic, Rochester, MN, USA

John C. Elfar, MD University of Rochester School of Medicine and Dentistry Center for Musculoskeletal Research, Rochester, NY, USA

Department of Orthopaedic Surgery, Hand and Upper Extremity and Sports Medicine, University of Rochester Medical Center, Rochester, NY, USA

Varun K. Gajendran, MD Department of Orthopaedic Surgery, MetroHealth Medical Center, Cleveland, OH, USA

Michael B. Geary, MD University of Rochester School of Medicine and Dentistry Center for Musculoskeletal Research, Rochester, NY, USA

Benjamin L. Gray, MD Department of Orthopaedic Surgery, University of Pennsylvania Health System, Pennsylvania Hospital, Philadelphia, PA, USA

Warren C. Hammert, MD Professor of Orthopaedic and Plastic Surgery, Chief, Division of Hand Surgery, Department of Orthopaedics and Rehabilitation, University of Rochester Medical Center, Rochester, NY, USA

Joshua Hudgens, MD Department of Orthopaedic Surgery, University of Michigan Health System, A. Alfred Taubman Health Care Center, Ann Arbor, MI, USA

J.M. Kirsch, MD Department of Orthopaedic Surgery, University of Michigan Health System, A. Alfred Taubman Health Care Center, Ann Arbor, MI, USA

Dawn M. LaPorte, MD Orthopaedic Surgery, Johns Hopkins University School of Medicine, Baltimore, MD, USA

Jeffrey N. Lawton, MD Department of Orthopaedic Surgery, University of Michigan Health System, A. Alfred Taubman Health Care Center, Ann Arbor, MI, USA

Laura W. Lewallen, MD Department of Orthopedic Surgery, Mayo Clinic, Rochester, MN, USA

Michael Maceroli, MD Resident Department of Orthopaedics and Rehabilitation, University of Rochester Medical Center, Rochester, NY, USA

Kevin J. Malone, MD Case Western Reserve University, Cleveland, OH, USA

Department of Orthopaedic Surgery, MetroHealth Medical Center, Cleveland, OH, USA

Andrew D. Markiewitz, MD Department of Orthopaedic Surgery, Trihealth Inc., Cincinnati, OH, USA

Kristofer S. Matullo, MD Department of Orthopaedic Surgery, St. Luke's University Health Network, Bethlehem, PA, USA

Eitan Melamed, MD Department of Plastic Surgery, Johns Hopkins Medical Center, Johns Hopkins Bayview Medical Center, Baltimore, MD, USA

Ryan A. Mlynarek, MD Department of Orthopaedic Surgery, University of Michigan Health System, A. Alfred Taubman Health Care Center, Ann Arbor, MI, USA

Nikhil R. Oak, MD Department of Orthopaedic Surgery, University of Michigan Health System, A. Alfred Taubman Health Care Center, Ann Arbor, MI, USA

Marco Rizzo, MD Department of Orthopedic Surgery, Mayo Clinic, Rochester, MN, USA

Rachel S. Rohde, MD Department of Orthopaedic Surgery, Oakland University William Beaumont School of Medicine, Michigan Orthopaedic Institute, Southfield, MI, USA

Mark C. Shreve, MD The CORE Institute, Novi, MI, USA

E.P. Tannenbaum, MD Department of Orthopaedic Surgery, University of Michigan Health System, A. Alfred Taubman Health Care Center, Ann Arbor, MI, USA

Jared Thomas, MD Department of Orthopaedic Surgery, University of Michigan Health System, A. Alfred Taubman Health Care Center, Ann Arbor, MI, USA

Jennifer Moriatis Wolf, MD Department of Orthopaedic Surgery, University of Connecticut Health Center, Farmington, CT, USA

Caroline N. Wolfe, MD Department of Orthopaedic Surgery, University of Michigan Health System, A. Alfred Taubman Health Care Center, Ann Arbor, MI, USA

Andy Zhu, MD Department of Orthopaedic Surgery, University of Michigan Health System, A. Alfred Taubman Health Care Center, Ann Arbor, MI, USA

Chapter 1
Treatment of Metaphyseal Distal Radius Fractures with a Volar Locking Plate

Rachel S. Rohde

Case

This 72-year-old right-hand dominant female fell onto her outstretched right hand. She was evaluated at a hospital based emergency center where she underwent closed reduction and splinting of a right distal radius fracture. At time of presentation, 10 days later, she denied any numbness or tingling and complained only of wrist pain and some pruritis from the cast material.

On physical examination, her right upper extremity was immobilized in a by then ill-fitting plaster splint extending to her proximal interphalangeal joints and encompassing her thumb in her palm. No neurovascular deficits were noted. Radiographs (Fig. 1.1) demonstrated a metaphyseal fracture of the right distal radius with complete dorsal displacement on the lateral view.

The chronicity of this fracture precluded an attempt at repeated closed reduction in the office. A discussion was had with the patient and her son regarding the risks and benefits of nonoperative and operative management, and a decision was made to proceed

R.S. Rohde, MD (✉)
Department of Orthopaedic Surgery, Oakland University William
Beaumont School of Medicine, Michigan Orthopaedic Institute, P.C.,
26025 Lahser Road, Southfield, MI 48033, USA
e-mail: rachel.rohde@beaumont.org

© Springer International Publishing Switzerland 2016   1
J.N. Lawton (ed.), *Distal Radius Fractures*,
DOI 10.1007/978-3-319-27489-8_1

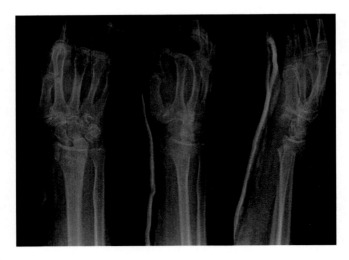

Fig. 1.1 Extra-articular distal radius fracture with poor alignment at first visit following closed reduction

with surgical management of the fracture. The patient underwent open reduction and internal fixation of the distal radius fracture using a volar distal radius locking plate the following day. Radiographs during her postoperative care demonstrated maintained alignment of her hardware and fracture (Fig. 1.2). She was issued a cock-up wrist splint and a prescription to start occupational hand therapy; she gradually pursued activities as tolerated.

The Literature

Indications

Management of distal radius fractures depends on fracture characteristics, patient factors, and surgeon preference. Although some extra-articular fractures can be reduced and maintained in the appropriate position until healing occurs, others are less stable and apt to lose reduction, prompting consideration of operative management.

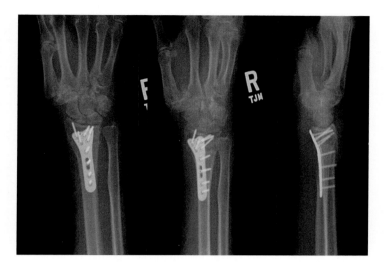

Fig. 1.2   Status post-ORIF distal radius fracture

Patient factors play a key role in determining management of metaphyseal distal radius fractures. Certainly, concomitant pathology such as multiple traumatic injuries and additional ipsilateral upper extremity soft tissue or bone injuries are potential indications for surgical treatment. Patients who are unable to tolerate prolonged immobilization for personal or professional reasons might benefit from the early mobilization allowed by internal fixation; although clinical outcomes are similar between many methods of treatment, internal fixation allows earlier discontinuation of immobilization, a requirement for certain occupational and avocational activities. With regard to its influence on fracture characteristics, patient age is one of the most reliable predictors of instability of these fractures [1]; early studies by McQueen et al. demonstrated that closed reduction of distal radius fractures in elderly patients failed in 53 of 60 wrists, 75 % within the first week after reduction [2]. It has been shown that distal radial fractures through osteopenic or osteoporotic bone are more likely to result in instability, malunion, and carpal malalignment [3]. Whether and when restoration of radiographic parameters is necessary for optimal functional outcome is beyond the scope of this chapter. Suffice it to say, that if between the surgeon and the patient, it is determined that maintained alignment is desired, then consideration should be given to open reduction and internal fixation. Finally, because closed treatment requires more frequent follow-up visits [4], patients for whom access to physicians for weekly follow-up is problematic might benefit from early surgical stabilization of the fracture.

Biomechanical Considerations

Much of the initial literature regarding the use of volar locking plates to treat distal radius fractures involved assessment of the biomechanics in extra-articular fractures created in cadaver specimens. Several studies have described the optimal approach to fixation. These screws are to be placed in a subchondral position [5] to support the articular surface. Penetration of the dorsal cortex can result in irritation and rupture of the extensor tendons, hence, the subchondral screws should not extend beyond the dorsal cortex; Liu et al. reported that using a screw that traverses 75 % of the depth of the distal radius is acceptable [6]. Although most volar locking plates have many holes for screw placement in the distal fragment, it has been shown that biomechanically, it is acceptable to use only half the screws [7, 8]; Mehling, however, reported that the construct is stronger with more screws [9].

Volar Plating Versus Other Surgical Options

The volar plate has been compared to other fixation methods for treatment of extra-articular and simple intra-articular distal radius fractures.

The use of external fixation and percutaneous pinning of these fractures preceded the introduction of the volar plate. A randomized trial of patients treated with volar locked plating versus external fixation for these fractures demonstrated improved outcomes of volar plating in the first 6 months; the discrepancy was minimal at

12 months [10]. Similarly, percutaneous Kirschner wire fixation demonstrated clinically and radiographically inferior results to volar plating for at least 6 months [11]; the follow-up was limited, so it is not known if the clinical differences persisted long term. Investigations comparing the outcomes following use of various techniques are ongoing.

More recently, the use of an intramedullary nail versus a volar plate led to better short-term (6 week) clinical outcomes, but no difference by 3 months; the nail use was associated with a risk of injury to the superficial branch of the radial nerve [12]. A different intramedullary device was investigated in a pilot study and demonstrated no differences from the volar plate; it is suggested that this might involve less soft tissue dissection than plate use [13]. In contrast, worse results were noted with the use of an intramedullary device versus a volar plate by another group [14]. The fractures for which intramedullary devices might be useful are more limited than those amenable to treatment with the volar plate, but this alternate device continues to be explored as an option to treat these extra-articular fractures.

Potential Complications

As with any surgery, open reduction and internal fixation using a volar plate is not without the standard risks of infection, nerve or blood vessel injury, malunion, nonunion, stiffness, and need for further procedures. Reported risks specific to the use of this hardware primarily address potential for tendon irritation and/or rupture. Extensor tendons can be irritated dorsally by even slightly prominent screws and tendon rupture can occur (Fig. 1.3) [15–20]. Flexor pollicis longus and flexor carpi radialis irritation or rupture also can occur secondary to irritation by the plate volarly [20–24]. Intra-articular screw placement, loss of reduction, extensor tenosynovitis, carpal tunnel syndrome, complex regional pain syndrome, screw loosening, and delayed union all have been observed [25]. The complication rate for volar plating of unstable distal radius fractures has been noted to range from less than 5 % [26] to as high as 48 % [27].

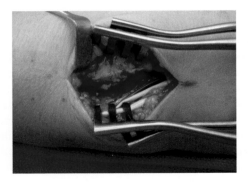

Fig. 1.3 Prominent dorsal screw tip that resulted in rupture of the extensor indicis proprius tendon

Postoperative Treatment

A benefit of the volar plate is that stable internal fixation can be achieved and early range of motion instituted. Although earlier range of motion does not appear to correlate with better long-term outcomes [28], this can be valuable to those who stand to lose significant productivity during the early months of recovery.

Case Review

Following loss of reduction in plaster immobilization, the fracture was not aligned appropriately to expect acceptable function. Therefore, a discussion was had with the patient regarding options for treatment. Although a second closed reduction could have been attempted in the operating room, the relative instability of this fracture already had been demonstrated. Closed reduction and percutaneous fixation was entertained as an option, but the patient had had difficulty tolerating the casting material already. In the author's hands, open reduction and internal fixation with a volar plate offered the most reliable opportunity to restore anatomy and function while minimizing complications. This also allowed early transition to a removable splint and initiation of range of motion exercises.

Tips/Tricks: Author's Opinion

A patient with a well-reduced extra-articular distal radius fracture should be counseled regarding the options for management. Maintenance of fracture position is monitored weekly for 3 weeks and then at 6 weeks post-fracture. If the reduction is not maintained, consideration is given to surgery. A frank discussion about the risks and benefits of operative and nonoperative treatment guides the patient and the surgeon to a mutually agreeable plan. Loss of reduction and intolerance of prolonged immobilization are the most common reasons for fixation to be recommended. Patients early in their treatment for whom prolonged immobilization poses a significant compromise to livelihood are considered for early fixation as well.

This surgery can be performed on an outpatient basis under a regional anesthetic for intra- and post-operative pain control. Alternatively, A general anesthetic may be a more appropriate option in some patients. In my experience, the use of an indwelling "pain pump" through which anesthesia is administered decreases post-operative pain and narcotic requirements.

I utilize the flexor carpi radialis tendon sheath approach and aim to align the volar cortex. When the fracture is difficult to maintain in a reduced position (as is usually the case in unstable fractures meriting fixation), a 0.0625 inch Kirschner wire can be inserted under fluoroscopic guidance through the radial styloid, across the fracture site, and into the metadiaphyseal bone. This provides provisional fixation for confirmation of reduction and then the plate is applied volarly. This often precludes styloid screw placement, so the K-wire is removed to complete fixation. I choose the implant according to specific needs of the fracture and the patient, and secondarily by my comfort with the system. I use screws to fix these fractures and am careful to aim the most ulnar distal screw slightly radially to avoid DRUJ penetration.

I generally use absorbable sutures and skin adhesive, both for cosmesis and because this alleviates any patient anxiety about having to have sutures removed at the first post-operative visit. Immobilization following surgery is primarily directed at comfort. A well-padded volar plaster splint is placed for comfort; this is discontinued approximately 1 week post-operatively and a pre-fabricated wrist cock-up splint is applied for comfort. The patient is allowed to remove this for motion exercises—with or without guidance of a hand therapist—and to shower.

Patients are advised that bones usually take 6–8 weeks to heal. They receive a prescription for hand therapy at the first postoperative visit and return in approximately 1 month for clinical and radiographic evaluation. Strengthening and gradual resumption of activities as tolerated begin if healing is progressing well at that time.

I do not routinely remove the hardware. Plate removal is considered if the patient experiences tendon irritation (or rupture) or other symptomatic hardware or if s/he has a peri-plate fracture and revision ORIF is performed.

References

1. Mackenney PJ, McQueen MM, Elton R. Prediction of instability in distal radial fractures. J Bone Joint Surg Am. 2006;88(9):1944–51.
2. Beumer A, McQueen MM. Fractures of the distal radius in low-demand elderly patients: closed reduction of no value in 53 of 60 wrists. Acta Orthop Scand. 2003;74(1):98–100.
3. Clayton RA, Gaston MS, Ralston SH, Court-Brown CM, Mcqueen MM. Association between decreased bone mineral density and severity of distal radial fractures. J Bone Joint Surg Am. 2009;91(3):613–9.
4. Lichtman DM, Bindra RR, Boyer MI, Putnam MD, Ring D, Slutsky DJ, Taras JS, Watters WC, Goldberg MJ, Keith M, Turkelson CM, Wies JL, Haralson RH, Boyer KM, Hitchcock K, Raymond L. AAOS clinical practice guideline summary: treatment of distal radius fractures. J Am Acad Orthop Surg. 2010;18:180–9.
5. Drobetz H, Bryant AL, Pokorny T, Spitaler R, Leixnering M, Jupiter JB. Volar fixed-angle plating of distal radius extension fractures: influence of plate position on secondary loss of reduction—a biomechanic study in a cadaveric model. J Hand Surg Am. 2006;31(4):615–22.

6. Liu X, Wu WD, Fang YF, Zhang MC, Huang WH. Biomechanical comparison of osteoporotic distal radius fractures fixed by distal locking screws with different length. PLoS One. 2014;9(7), e103371.
7. Crosby SN, Fletcher ND, Yap ER, Lee DH. The mechanical stability of extra-articular distal radius fractures with respect to the number of screws securing the distal fragment. J Hand Surg Am. 2013;38(6):1097–105.
8. Moss DP, Means Jr KR, Parks BG, Forthman CL. A biomechanical comparison of volar locked plating of intra-articular distal radius fractures: use of 4 versus 7 screws for distal fixation. J Hand Surg Am. 2011;36(12): 1907–11.
9. Mehling I, Müller LP, Delinsky K, Mehler D, Burkhart KJ, Rommens PM. Number and locations of screw fixation for volar fixed-angle plating of distal radius fractures: biomechanical study. J Hand Surg Am. 2010;35(6):885–91.
10. Wilcke MK, Abbaszadegan H, Adolphson PY. Wrist function recovers more rapidly after volar locked plating than after external fixation but the outcomes are similar after 1 year. Acta Orthop. 2011;82(1):76–81.
11. McFadyen I, Field J, McCann P, Ward J, Nicol S, Curwen C. Should unstable extra-articular distal radial fractures be treated with fixed-angle volar-locked plates or percutaneous Kirschner wires? A prospective randomised controlled trial. Injury. 2011;42(2):162–6.
12. Safi A, Hart R, Těknědžjan B, Kozák T. Treatment of extra-articular and simple articular distal radial fractures with intramedullary nail versus volar locking plate. J Hand Surg Eur. 2013;38(7):774–9.
13. Zehir S, Calbiyik M, Zehir R, Ipek D. Intramedullary repair device against volar plating in the reconstruction of extra-articular and simple articular distal radius fractures; a randomized pilot study. Int Orthop. 2014;38(8): 1655–60.
14. Chappuis J, Bouté P, Putz P. Dorsally displaced extra-articular distal radius fractures fixation: Dorsal IM nailing versus volar plating. A randomized controlled trial. Orthop Traumatol Surg Res. 2011;97(5): 471–8.
15. Al-Rashid M, Theivendran K, Craigen MA. Delayed ruptures of the extensor tendon secondary to the use of volar locking compression plates for distal radial fractures. J Bone Joint Surg Br. 2006;88:1610–2.
16. Benson EC, DeCarvalho A, Mikola EA, Veitch JM, Moneim MS. Two potential causes of EPL rupture after distal radius volar plate fixation. Clin Orthop Relat Res. 2006;451:218–22.
17. Engkvist O, Lundborg G. Rupture of the extensor pollicis longus tendon after fracture of the lower end of the radius: a clinical and microangiographic study. Hand. 1979;11:76–86.
18. Failla JM, Koniuch MP, Moed BR. Extensor pollicis longus rupture at the tip of a prominent fixation screw: report of three cases. J Hand Surg Am. 1993;18:648–51.
19. Wong-Chung J, Quinlan W. Rupture of extensor pollicis longus following fixation of a distal radius fracture. Injury. 1989;20:375–6.

20. Rozental TD, Beredjiklian PK, Bozentka DJ. Functional outcome and complications following two types of dorsal plating for unstable fractures of the distal part of the radius. J Bone Joint Surg Am. 2003;85:1956–60.

21. Bell JS, Wollstein R, Citron ND. Rupture of flexor pollicis longus tendon: a complication of volar plating of the distal radius. J Bone Joint Surg Br. 1998;80:225–6.

22. DiMatteo L, Wolf JM. Flexor carpi radialis tendon rupture as a complication of a closed distal radius fracture: a case report. J Hand Surg Am. 2007;32: 818–20.

23. Klug RA, Press CM, Gonzalez MH. Rupture of the flexor pollicis longus tendon after volar fixed-angle plating of a distal radius fracture: a case report. J Hand Surg Am. 2007;32:984–8.

24. Koo SC, Ho ST. Delayed rupture of the flexor pollicis longus tendon after volar plating of the distal radius. Hand Surg. 2006;11:67–70.

25. Arora R, Lutz M, Hennerbichler A, Krappinger D, Espen D, Gabi M. Complications following internal fixation of unstable distal radius fracture with a palmar locking-plate. J Orthop Trauma. 2007;21(5):316–22.

26. Fok MWM, Klausmeyer MA, Fernandez DL, Orbay JL, Bergada AL. Volar plate fixation of intra-articular distal radius fractures: a retrospective study. J Wrist Surg. 2013;2(3):247–54.

27. Knight D, Hajducka C, Will E, McQueen M. Locked volar plating for unstable distal radial fractures: clinical and radiological outcomes. Injury. 2010;41(2):184–9.

28. Lozano-Calderon SA, Souer S, Mudgal C, Jupiter JB, Ring D. Wrist mobilization following volar plate fixation of fractures of the distal part of the radius. J Bone Joint Surg Am. 2008;90:1297–304.

Chapter 2
Volar Plate/Hook Pin for Volar Lunate Facet Fragment

Michael Maceroli and Warren C. Hammert

Case Presentation

A 50-year-old right-hand dominant businessman sustained multiple injuries when his snowmobile collided with a tree while traveling at approximately 45 mph. He was evaluated at a referral institution, where he was diagnosed with a right scapula fracture, multiple rib fractures, and a right distal radius fracture. A splint was placed on the right wrist without fracture manipulation; and he presented to our office 4 days after the initial trauma for management of the wrist injury. In addition to pain in the right wrist the patient reported numbness and tingling in the median nerve distribution in the hand.

M. Maceroli, MD
Resident, Department of Orthopaedics and Rehabilitation,
University of Rochester Medical Center, 601 Elmwood Ave.,
Box 665, Rochester, NY 14642, USA
e-mail: Michael_Maceroli@urmc.rochester.edu

W.C. Hammert, MD (✉)
Professor of Orthopaedic and Plastic Surgery, Chief, Division of Hand Surgery, Department of Orthopaedics and Rehabilitation,
University of Rochester Medical Center, Rochester, NY 14642, USA
e-mail: Warren_Hammert@URMC.Rochester.edu

© Springer International Publishing Switzerland 2016   11
J.N. Lawton (ed.), *Distal Radius Fractures*,
DOI 10.1007/978-3-319-27489-8_2

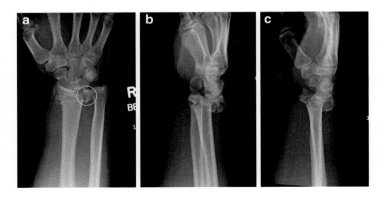

Fig. 2.1 Preoperative radiographs of 50-year-old male right wrist demonstrating a dorsally displaced, comminuted, intra-articular distal radius fracture. (**a**) AP radiograph clearly shows the displaced volar lunate facet fragment (*white circle*). (**b** and **c**) Oblique and lateral radiographs show the dorsal displacement and intra-articular comminution

PA, lateral, and oblique radiographs of the right wrist demonstrate a dorsally displaced, comminuted intra-articular distal radius fracture (Fig. 2.1). There is a radial styloid fragment, a separate volar lunate facet fragment, as well as dorsal comminution. The teardrop angle measure on the lateral projection is 50° (Fig. 2.2).

The patient elected to proceed with surgical management of this fracture. The procedure was performed under brachial plexus nerve block with sedation anesthesia.

A 6 cm longitudinal incision was made in the volar wrist, using an extended flexor carpi radialis (FCR) approach. A trans-FCR carpal tunnel release was performed [1] and the interval between the FCR and the radial artery was developed and opened, retracting the flexor tendons and median nerve in an ulnar direction to expose the pronator quadratus. This was elevated off the radius to expose the fracture and distal shaft. The brachioradialis was released from its insertion on the radial styloid fragments—protecting the first dorsal compartment tendons.

The dorsal scar was released with pronation of the proximal fragment and preliminary reduction of the radial styloid, scaphoid facet fragment, and the volar lunate facet fragment was achieved

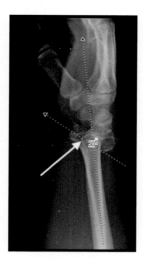

Fig. 2.2 Preoperative lateral wrist radiograph demonstrating the teardrop angle of 50°. The volar lunate facet can be identified as a teardrop shaped area on the lateral wrist plain radiograph (*white arrow*). The teardrop angle is a described radiographic measurement formed between a line along the longitudinal radial axis and the central axis of the teardrop itself

and provisionally held with Kirschner (K) wires. The lunate facet fragment was small and the fracture was at the level of the watershed line. A Geminus plate (Skeletal Dynamics, Miami, FL) was placed on the volar surface of the radius and provisionally fixed with one proximal shaft screw and distal K wires. After fluoroscopic confirmation of appropriate plate position, the styloid and scaphoid facets were supported with locking pegs. The lunate facet fragment was supported with two smooth locking pegs. Due to the distal fracture location of the lunate facet fragment, a hook plate attachment was secured to the volar plate supporting the lunate facet fragment and providing volar support for the carpus through attachment of the short radiolunate ligament. The plate was then secured to the radial shaft with six cortices of fixation. This distal radioulnar joint (DRUJ) was assessed and felt to be stable. The pronator quadratus was repaired and the wound was closed in layers. A short arm volar plaster splint was applied.

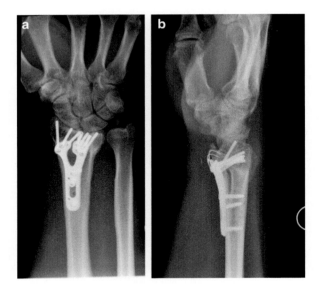

Fig. 2.3 PA (**a**) and lateral (**b**) right wrist radiographs at 8 months postoperative demonstrating the positioning of the hook plate attachment, anatomic fracture reduction, and maintenance of the radiocarpal articulation

The patient was transitioned to a short arm cast due to the volar lunate facet fragment, but continued working on finger and elbow motion. At 4 weeks, he was transitioned to a removable orthosis and began a formal hand therapy and home exercise program focusing on wrist and forearm motion. His fracture healed without loss of reduction (Fig. 2.3). The patient demonstrated excellent clinical range of motion at last follow-up (Fig. 2.4) with details of motion presented in Table 2.1. The patient was able to return to work and all other activities without limitations or difficulty.

Review of the Literature

Intra-articular fractures of the distal radius that include a separate coronal plane fragment at the volar lunate facet represent a difficult subset of fractures. They are often challenging to identify on

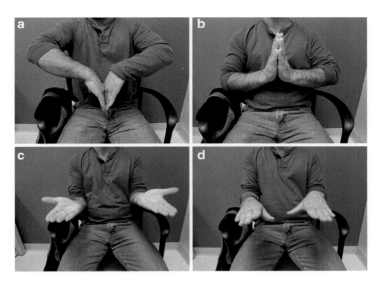

Fig. 2.4 Clinical photographs demonstrating wrist range of motion at 8 months following surgery. (**a**) Wrist flexion, (**b**) wrist extension, (**c**) supination, and (**d**) pronation

Table 2.1 Wrist range of motion at 8-month follow-up

	Right	Left
Flexion	45	50
Extension	30	50
Radial deviation	25	25
Ulnar deviation	30	40
Pronation	70	80
Supination	60	70

initial radiographs. Furthermore, gaining adequate fixation in an often small, unstable lunate facet fragment is deceivingly difficult to achieve with standard volar plating techniques. Loss of fixation in the volar lunate facet fragment can result in volar subluxation of the carpus. Malunion in this position has potentially devastating functional ramifications.

The volar lunate facet fragment, as originally described by Melone, is the origin of the volar radiolunate ligaments [2, 3]. The lunate facet region slopes volarly at the attachment of the radiolunate ligaments. According to radiographic studies, this area projects an average of 3 mm anterior to the relatively flat volar radius [4]. This anatomic consideration prevents a plate from lying flat over the volar lunate facet fragment and weakens the buttress effect of the locked volar plate. Furthermore, the volar lunate fragment is often small in comparison to the larger radial styloid and dorsal articular fragments. The surgeon may only be able to achieve a single screw transfixing the volar lunate facet fragment leading to inadequate stability and failure [5].

Multiple case series have highlighted distal radius fracture failure following inadequate fixation of the volar lunate facet, resulting in volar subluxation of the carpus [3, 5–7]. This highlights the stabilizing effect the lunate facet has on the carpus and the devastating deformity that occurs after fixation failure — with volar escape of the lunate and carpal subluxation.

Harness et al. reported on seven cases of distal radius fracture failure due to inadequate fixation of the volar lunate facet [3]. In this study, all patients were initially treated with volar plating and all postoperative radiographs demonstrated anatomic reduction of the volar fragments. After initiation of active wrist range of motion all seven patients had loss of reduction of the volar lunate facet, four of which resulted in radiocarpal subluxation. These patients suffered from reduced wrist range of motion and grip strength as compared to their uninjured, contralateral side [3]. These deficits remained constant even after revision surgery, emphasizing the importance of early recognition and fixation of the lunate facet fragment during the index procedure.

Despite the aforementioned case series, not all peri-articular distal radius fractures with separate volar lunate facet fragments are destined to fail. Beck et al. evaluated radiographic features in 52 volar shear pattern distal radius fractures [6]. Seven of the 52 fractures went on to failure after initial fixation. The authors reported that preoperative lunate facet subsidence greater than 5 mm and/or length of the volar cortex less than 15 mm were associated with failure following locked volar plating [6]. They also reported that the presence of separate scaphoid and lunate facet fragments was a risk factor for failure. Based on these results, the treating surgeon should employ alternatives or adjuncts to locked volar plating alone when dealing with small, displaced lunate facet fragments.

When treating volar shear articular fractures of the distal radius, the surgeon must first determine the presence of a separate lunate facet fragment. When diagnosed, adequate exposure is required to visualize the radioulnar articulation to perform anatomic reduction. Various fixation techniques can then be employed to either improve the volar plate buttress effect or increase the number of fixation points, ensuring capture of the fragment.

Early diagnosis of the displaced volar lunate facet fragment is arguably the most important step in the treatment of this distal radius fracture subset. The volar lunate facet can be identified as a teardrop shaped area on the lateral wrist plain radiograph [8]. The teardrop angle is a described radiographic measurement formed between a line along the longitudinal radial axis and the central axis of the teardrop itself [8]. Fujitani et al. demonstrated statistically notable correlation to articular stepoff with a teardrop angle of less than 45° with near perfect interobserver and intraobserver reliability [9]. In addition, computed tomography (CT) imaging can be helpful for identifying the extent of articular involvement, fragment size, and comminution [10].

During exposure, care must be taken to expose the distal and ulnar most aspect of the volar radius (Fig. 2.5). After adequate

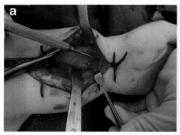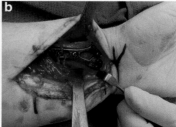

Fig. 2.5 Clinical photograph demonstrating exposure of the volar lunate facet portion of the radius before (**a**—probe is pointing to volar lunate facet) and after securing volar locked plate (**b**)

exposure, the lunate facet fragment can be provisionally reduced prior to final implant selection and fixation. There are multiple described methods for definitive fixation that should be in the operating surgeon's armamentarium when planning to treat the volar lunate facet fracture.

Chin and Jupiter described the wire-loop fixation method for treatment of volar sided articular distal radius fractures [11]. In this method the radial styloid fragment is reduced by closed means and transfixed with 1 or 2, 0.062-inch K wires. The volar lunate facet fragment is then reduced through an ulnar sided approach to the radius between the ulnar neurovascular bundle and the flexor tendons. The fragment is reduced and a 2.5 mm drill is used to make two cortical holes in the radial metaphysis 1 cm proximal to the fracture. A 19-gauge wire is passed through the drill holes, and then shuttled underneath the volar capsule just distal to the fracture, and finally the wire is manually tensioned. In the author's initial case series, all four patients treated in this fashion achieved pain-free fracture union and 75 % regained equivalent wrist range of motion compared to the contralateral, uninjured side [11].

The addition of a spring wire construct to a standard volar locked radius plate is another technique to apply concentrated points of fixation to the small, lunate facet fragment. After reduction of the lunate facet, a 0.035-inch K wire is advanced from the volar lip of the fragment, across the fracture and seated in the proximal, dorsal cortex. The wire is then bent to match the contour of the volar radius and the standard volar plate is placed overtop, fixing the remainder of the fracture. A case series of nine patients treated in this fashion all went on to complete healing and none required hardware removal [12]. These patients achieved a mean 46° wrist flexion, 51° wrist extension, 80° supination, 68° pronation, and an average Patient Rated Wrist Evaluation (PRWE) score of 17 [12].

Volar locked plates with variable angle screws can often achieve some fixation in the lunate facet fragment; however, with smaller fragments, only one transfixing screw may be possible [13]. This is suboptimal unless the volar plate applies a buttress effect on the fragment. Unfortunately, the lunate facet fragment location often necessitates placing the plate distal and volar to the watershed line, risking flexor tendon irritation and rupture [14]. If the volar plate is applied in this fashion, it is recommended to remove the plate and screw construct after fracture healing [14].

Clearly there are drawbacks to traditional volar plate application to displaced lunate facet fragments. Fortunately, new innovations in volar plate technology allow for fragment specific fixation. The Geminus (Skeletal Dynamics, Miami, FL) plates offer separate limbs to support the scaphoid and lunate fossae and can be contoured to patient specific anatomy. This allows for maximum fixation in the volar lunate facet. These plates also offer a hook plate attachment that secures to the plate and extends over the lunate facet fragment for extra support. Additionally, other fragment specific fixation systems offer multiple plating options to accommodate various peri-articular patterns. Saw et al. reviewed 21 cases treated with fragment specific fixation and reported no loss of reduction at minimum 6-month follow-up [15]. The mean range of wrist and forearm motion was 50° flexion, 63° extension, and supination-pronation arc of 149° [15].

When patients present early with failure after volar plating due to displacement of the volar lunate facet, the surgeon may attempt revision open reduction and internal fixation. The key to reduction is reestablishing the volar ulnar cortical edge, anatomically reducing the facet, and applying an ulnar column buttress plate [5], or other means to stabilize the lunate facet fragment. If the patient presents late with a malunion, excellent functional outcomes have resulted from corrective intra-articular osteotomy surgery [16].

Tips and Tricks

- Identification of the displaced volar lunate facet fragment using the teardrop angle or preoperative CT imaging to allow for appropriate surgical planning.
- Place the volar locked plate as ulnar as possible to allow maximum screw fixation in the fragment while avoiding penetration of the sigmoid notch. The plate should be proximal to the watershed line and the fracture should be reduced/in contact with the plate.

- Clearly visualize the fracture line of the lunate facet fragment. It is common for the rim of the plate to cover the fracture line, giving the surgeon the false sense of stabilization of the fragment as the screw or peg may be in the fracture.
- New generation volar plates allow fragment specific contouring of the scaphoid and lunate facet fragments to direct variable angle screws as needed into the fractures. These still may not be able to secure the fragment and care must be taken to ensure the variable angle screw does not penetrate the articular surface of the radiocarpal or distal radial ulnar joints.
- Use of a hook plate attachment provides additional points of fixation supporting the lunate facet fragment with a low-profile implant.
- A tension band construct can supplement a standard volar plate using #2 FiberWire (Arthrex, Naples, FL). The suture can be passed through bone tunnels proximal to the fracture fragment and then tied to the volar capsule.
- Fluoroscopy should be used to confirm appropriate position of distal pegs/screws just below the level of the subchondral bone and that they do not penetrate the radial carpal joint or DRUJ.
- Following stabilization, the surgeon should check to ensure that the carpus does not sublux with volar directed force and should assess for DRUJ instability by stressing the dorsal and volar radial ulnar ligaments. If instability at either the radiocarpal or distal radial ulnar joint is present, it should be addressed prior to leaving the operating room.

References

1. Pensy RA, Brunton LM, Parks BG, Higgins JP, Chhabra AB. Single-incision extensile volar approach to the distal radius and concurrent carpal tunnel release: cadaveric study. J Hand Surg Am. 2010;35(2):217–22.
2. Melone CP. Articular fractures of the distal radius. Orthop Clin North Am. 1984;15(2):217–36.
3. Harness NG, Jupiter JB, Orbay JL, Raskin KB, Fernandez DL. Loss of fixation of the volar lunate facet fragment in fractures of the distal part of the radius. J Bone Joint Surg Am. 2004;86-A(9):1900–8.

4. Andermahr J, Lozano-Calderon S, Trafton T, Crisco JJ, Ring D. The volar extension of the lunate facet of the distal radius: a quantitative anatomic study. J Hand Surg Am. 2006;31(6):892–5.
5. Kitay A, Mudgal C. Volar carpal subluxation following lunate facet fracture. J Hand Surg Am. 2014;39(11):2335–41.
6. Beck JD, Harness NG, Spencer HT. Volar plate fixation failure for volar shearing distal radius fractures with small lunate facet fragments. J Hand Surg Am. 2014;39(4):670–8.
7. Apergis E, Darmanis S, Theodoratos G, Maris J. Beware of the ulno-palmar distal radial fragment. J Hand Surg Br. 2002;27(2):139–45.
8. Medoff RJ. Essential radiographic evaluation for distal radius fractures. Hand Clin. 2005;21(3):279–88.
9. Fujitani R, Omokawa S, Iida A, Santo S, Tanaka Y. Reliability and clinical importance of teardrop angle measurement in intra-articular distal radius fracture. J Hand Surg Am. 2012;37(3):454–9.
10. Souer JS, Wiggers J, Ring D. Quantitative 3-dimensional computed tomography measurement of volar shearing fractures of the distal radius. J Hand Surg Am. 2011;36(4):599–603.
11. Chin KR, Jupiter JB. Wire-loop fixation of volar displaced osteochondral fractures of the distal radius. J Hand Surg Am. 1999;24(3):525–33.
12. Moore AM, Dennison DG. Distal radius fractures and the volar lunate facet fragment: Kirschner wire fixation in addition to volar-locked plating. Hand (N Y). 2014;9(2):230–6.
13. Hart A, Collins M, Chhatwal D, Steffen T, Harvey EJ, Martineau PA. Can the use of variable-angle volar locking plates compensate for suboptimal plate positioning in unstable distal radius fractures? a biomechanical study. J Orthop Trauma. 2015;29:e1–6.
14. Kitay A, Swanstrom M, Schreiber JJ, et al. Volar plate position and flexor tendon rupture following distal radius fracture fixation. J Hand Surg Am. 2013;38(6):1091–6.
15. Saw N, Roberts C, Cutbush K, Hodder M, Couzens G, Ross M. Early experience with the TriMed fragment-specific fracture fixation system in intraarticular distal radius fractures. J Hand Surg Eur Vol. 2008;33(1):53–8.
16. Ruch DS, Wray WH, Papadonikolakis A, Richard MJ, Leversedge FJ, Goldner RD. Corrective osteotomy for isolated malunion of the palmar lunate facet in distal radius fractures. J Hand Surg Am. 2010;35(11):1779–86.

Chapter 3
Volar Locking Plate + Dorsal-Ulnar Plate

Michael Darowish

Case Examples

Patient 1

A 46-year-old woman sustained a comminuted right distal radius fracture in a motorcycle accident (Fig. 3.1a, b). Fixation was performed with a volar plate, and intraoperative radiographs demonstrated acceptable articular surface alignment (Fig. 3.2a, b). The scapholunate distance was noted to be widened; however, comparision to older radiographs confirmed this to be a chronic ligamentous injury, and not an acute tear. At her postoperative appointment, there was concern for the alignment of the lunate fossa (Fig. 3.3); and a CT scan obtained showed that the articular surface had settled around the distal screws due to inadequate support (Fig. 3.4a, b). Revision of the fixation with a dorsal-ulnar plate to better buttress the articular surface was performed (Fig. 3.5a, b).

M. Darowish, MD (✉)
Department of Orthopaedic Surgery, Penn State Milton S. Hershey Medical Center, 30 Hope Drive, P.O. Box 859, Hershey 17033, PA, USA
e-mail: mdarowish@hmc.psu.edu

© Springer International Publishing Switzerland 2016
J.N. Lawton (ed.), *Distal Radius Fractures*,
DOI 10.1007/978-3-319-27489-8_3

23

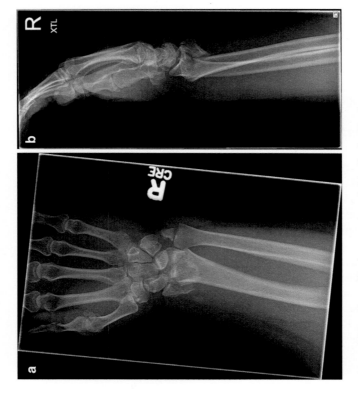

Fig. 3.1 Initial PA (**a**) and lateral (**b**) radiographs of a comminuted right distal radius fracture

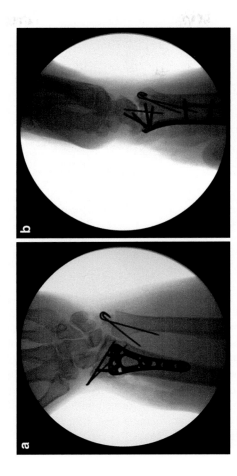

Fig. 3.2 Intraoperative PA (**a**) and lateral (**b**) radiographs. Volar locking plate fixation was performed, with supplemental K-wires in the radial styloid, as only one screw could be placed in the styloid fragment. The ulnar styloid was fixed with K-wires, as the DRUJ was unstable until this was performed. The scapholunate distance was noted to be widened; however, comparision to older radiographs confirmed this to be a chronic ligamentous injury, and not an acute tear

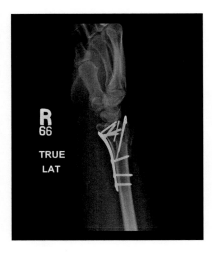

Fig. 3.3 Postoperative lateral radiograph. Based on this film, there was concern for loss of reduction and fixation of the articular surface of the dorsal-ulnar distal radius

Patient 2

A 51-year-old man sustained a comminuted left distal radius fracture. Preoperative CT scan showed the lunate facet to be a separate fragment from the remainder of the articular surface (Fig. 3.6a, b). Initial fixation was performed with a volar plate; the distal radius seemed stable intraoperatively (Fig. 3.7a, b). However, on follow-up radiographs, the dorsal-ulnar fragment displaced dorsally, and the carpus subluxated or escaped dorsally with the fragment (Fig. 3.8). Revision fixation was performed with a dorsal plate to better capture the dorsal-ulnar fragment (Fig. 3.9a, b). The fracture went on to uneventful healing.

Introduction

Occasionally, one is confronted with a distal radius fracture in which there is dorsal or articular surface comminution in combination with loss of reduction. With the advent of locking volar plates,

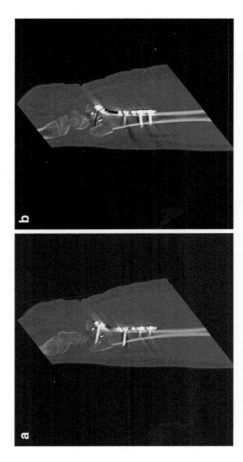

Fig. 3.4 Postoperative CT scan slices demonstrating settling of the articular surface around the distal screw from the volar plate and possible dorsal displacement of the dorsal cortex

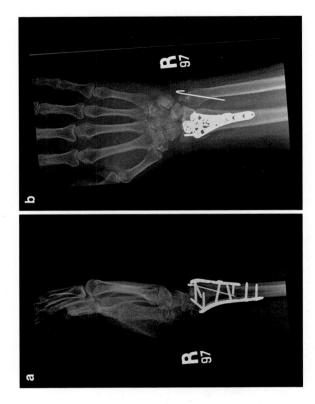

Fig. 3.5 Lateral (**a**) and PA (**b**) views status-post revision fixation with placement of a dorsal-ulnar plate. Note the restoration of alignment and improved buttressing of the ulnar aspect of the articular surface

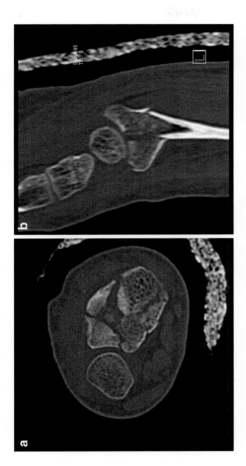

Fig. 3.6 Preoperative axial (**a**) and sagittal (**b**) CT scans of a comminuted distal radius fracture. Note the separate dorsal-ulnar fragment containing portions of both the lunate facet articular surface and sigmoid notch articular surface

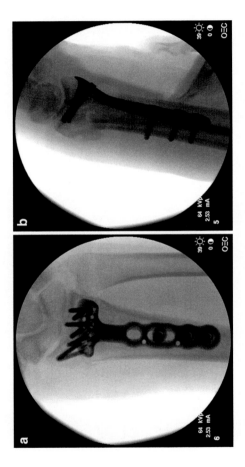

Fig. 3.7 Intraoperative PA (**a**) and lateral (**b**) radiographs during initial fixation with volar locking plate

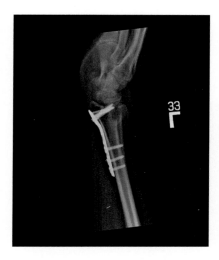

Fig. 3.8 Postoperative lateral radiograph demonstrating escape of the dorsal-ulnar fragment and posterior displacement of the lunate

many of these fractures are able to be adequately stabilized from a volar approach only. However, some fractures require supplemental fixation of this dorsal fragment to prevent escape of the dorsal-ulnar fragment, and with it, subluxation of the carpus. Additionally, some more comminuted fractures require more subchondral support of the articular surface than a volar plate can provide on its own. This chapter will describe this combined fixation technique.

Indications

There are two primary indications for combined volar and dorsal-ulnar fixation. The first is if the dorsal-ulnar fragment of the distal radius (including the lunate fossa and sigmoid notch) is a separate fragment from the remainder of the articular surface and is not adequately captured by the distal screws of a volar plate (as demonstrated in the case of Patient 2). The second indication is depression or comminution of the articular surface which cannot

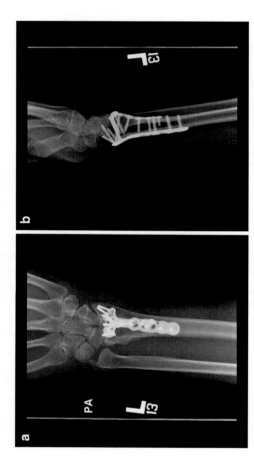

Fig. 3.9 PA (**a**) and lateral (**b**) radiographs demonstrating a healed fracture status-post revision fixation with a dorsal-ulnar plate, which restored alignment of the distal radius and returned the carpus to anatomic relationship with the distal radius

be adequately buttressed by the distal screws of a volar plate alone (as demonstrated in the case of Patient 1).

Unfortunately, many of these fracture patterns are not immediately obvious on presentation, and can be missed intraoperatively as well. Thus one must maintain a high index of suspicion preoperatively and mandate a good quality lateral film, as this subtlety can be easily overlooked on a slightly oblique "lateral" radiograph. Even when identified, it can seem that these fragments are stabilized with volar fixation. Even intraoperative stressing of the fracture cannot adequately predict the stability of fixation. Often, these are recognized on postoperative radiographs, requiring revision fixation. A high index of suspicion and low threshold of adding a dorsal plate are required by the physician to identify and treat these fractures adequately at the index procedure.

Technique

The technique of volar plating is covered extensively throughout this text. However, I have found several details which markedly help this procedure. The patient is positioned supine with an upper arm tourniquet. General and/or regional anesthesia is used.

A mini C-arm is utilized for intraoperative fluoroscopy. I find it helpful to position the fluoroscope parallel with the floor. By doing so, both sides of the fluoroscope are kept sterile, and magnification and radiation scatter are minimized by allowing the hand to be positioned directly onto the receiver, taking care to avoid contamination by inadvertently poking through the sterile cover with any K-wires.

I utilize the distal portion of the anterior approach of Henry [1], dissecting the radial artery along its length and mobilizing it radially. Several small perforating branches must be coagulated with bipolar electrocautery in order to adequately mobilize the artery. The floor of the radial artery sheath is incised. Digital dissection is then used to mobilize the flexor carpi radialis (FCR) and the carpal tunnel contents ulnarly. Occasionally there are vertical fascial bands which must be divided to adequately expose the pronator quadratus (PQ).

In many cases, the brachioradialis (BR) tendon needs to be released to improve the ability of the surgeon to restore radial height and inclination. To safely accomplish this, a small opening is made into the first dorsal compartment along the radial aspect of the distal radius at or distal to the fracture line. The abductor pollicis longus (APL) and extensor pollicis brevis (EPB) are identified and retracted radially. The BR is identified deep to these tendons in the floor of the first compartment. With the APL and EPB tendons protected, the BR can be sharply released from the distal fragment, improving the surgeon's ability to mobilize the distal radial fragment into a reduced position, with no meaningful loss of function [2, 3].

The fascia of the PQ is incised in an L-shape along the distal and radial aspects, leaving a cuff of tissue to repair the fascia at the conclusion of the case. The muscle fibers of the PQ are elevated with a periosteal elevator. The fracture can be directly visualized and reduced. Because the bone volarly is typically stronger and less comminuted than dorsally, provisional reduction and judgement of length and inclination is more easily accomplished from this approach [4]. Kirschner wires (K-wires) are used to temporarily hold the fracture in a reduced position. A volar plate is then positioned on the distal radius and held with K-wires. Fixation then proceeds either distally-to-proximally, which allows the plate to be utilized to restore volar tilt; or proximally-to-distally, which provides a volar butress to which reduction and fixation can be based. If proximal-to-distal fixation is utilized, care must be used in selecting distal fixation, as locking screws will not help to achieve reduction, only stabilizing whatever reduction has been obtained prior to their insertion.

In cases where dorsal plating is used in combination with volar plating, the order of fixation of the articular surface may be variable. If the dorsal plate is being used as purely supplementation to the volar fixation, then it can be applied later; however, in most cases, where the dorsal plate is primary fixation of a dorsal-ulnar fragment or to buttress a comminuted articular surface, it is helpful to apply the dorsal plate before placement of the distal screws of the volar plate. Additionally, if intraarticular visualization is required for adequate reduction of the fracture, the dorsal approach and fixation should be performed prior to distal fixation volarly.

The dorsal plate is applied through a dorsal incision centered on the radial shaft. Because of dorsal comminution, Lister's tubercle is often not palpable, and fluoroscopic localization is required for incision placement. The extensor pollicis longus (EPL) is identified and released from the third compartment. The fourth compartment tendons (extensor digitorum communis (EDC) and extensor indicis proprius (EIP)) are elevated ulnarly. At this point, the surgeon must decide if intraarticular visualization through an arthrotomy is necessary. If the articular surface needs to be directly observed for reduction or if other intraarticular pathology needs to be addressed simultaneously (e.g., scapholunate dissociation), an arthrotomy can be created and the surface reduced under direct visualization. If intraarticular visualization is not necessary, the wrist capsule can be left intact [5].

The dorsal-ulnar plate is positioned and held in place with K-wires. The specific plate selected is per surgeon preference; the metal used should be compatible with the volar plating system to prevent galvanic corrosion; the plate shape (straight, T, or L-shaped) should be chosen to match the fracture pattern and function required of the plate. Care must be taken to directly appose the plate to the bone; even with modern low-profile plates, irritation, abrasion, or rupture of the extensor tendons can occur with poorly positioned plates.

Because the dorsal rim is more distal than the volar rim, the dorsal plate may appear to be intraarticular on AP radiographs; careful examination both *in vivo* intraoperatively and on lateral radiographs (both standard lateral and radial inclined lateral views) is necessary to ensure appropriate positioning of the plate on the dorsal distal radius and extraarticular subchondral placement of the distal screws. In cases where both volar and dorsal plating are utilized, the availability of variable angle screws may be beneficial to allow multiple screws to be placed in a small anatomic area without impinging on one another. If necessary, bone grafting to support the chondral surface can be accomplished through the dorsal fracture site with autograft, allograft, or bone substitute at the surgeon's preference.

After appropriate fluoroscopic images are obtained, closure is by standard means. I leave the EPL transposed above the extensor retinaculum with a so-called subcutaneous pulley. If possible, subperiosteal dissection of the fourth dorsal compartment will allow interposed soft tissue between the dorsal plate and extensor tendons. Volarly, I try to repair the PQ over the plate, accepting that in many cases this is not possible, and has little benefit functionally [6, 7]. However, the benefit of interposing soft tissue between the plate and the flexor tendons makes it worth the attempt.

Following fixation of the distal radius, the DRUJ must be checked for stability in pronation, supination, and neutral forearm rotation, and appropriate stabilization of any instability must be performed. Even in cases of apparent DRUJ stability, I immobilize the forearm in supination for the first 10 days postoperatively and immediately initiate finger range of motion exercises. I then convert to a removable short arm splint, adding forearm rotation, but typically do not initiate wrist ROM until 6 weeks postoperatively.

References

1. Chapter 4: The forearm. In: Hoppenfeld S, deBoer P, editors. Surgical exposures in orthopaedics: the anatomic approach. 3rd ed. Philadelphia: Lippincott Williams & Wilkins; 2003.
2. Koh S, Andersen CR, Buford Jr WL, Patterson RM, Viegas SF. Anatomy of the distal brachioradialis and its potential relationship to distal radius fracture. J Hand Surg Am. 2006;31(1):2–8.
3. Irrell TF, Franko OI, Bhola S, Hentzen ER, Abrams RA, Lieber RL. Functional consequence of distal brachioradialis tendon release: a biomechanical study. J Hand Surg. 2013;38A:920–6.
4. Ring D, Prommersburger K, Jupiter JB. Volar plate fixation of complex fractures of the distal part of the radius: surgical technique. J Bone Joint Surg (Am). 2005;87-A:195–212.
5. Ilyas AM. Surgical approaches to the distal radius. Hand. 2011;6(1):8–17.
6. Hershman SH, Immerman I, Bechtel C, Lekic N, Paksima N, Egol KA. The effects of pronator quadratus repair on outcomes after volar plating of distal radius fractures. J Orthop Trauma. 2013;27(3):130–3.
7. Tosti R, Ilyas AM. Prospective evaluation of pronator quadratus repair following volar plate fixation of distal radius fractures. J Hand Surg Am. 2013;38(9):1678–84.

Chapter 4
Volar Locking Plate and Radial Styloid Plating

Jeffrey N. Lawton and Joshua Hudgens

Case History

A 47-year-old right-hand dominant construction worker fell approximately 12 feet from a scaffold sustaining an isolated injury of his left wrist. In addition to the closed, comminuted left distal radius fracture (Fig. 4.1a–c) he also sustained an acute carpal tunnel syndrome and a hand compartment syndrome. He underwent carpal tunnel release, hand fasciotomies, and open reduction internal fixation (ORIF) of his distal radius fracture. ORIF was performed with a volar locking plate and radial styloid plate given the fracture pattern, demonstrating a large and comminuted radial styloid fragment (Fig. 4.2a, b). Following ORIF, he was found to have gross instability of his distal radioulnar joint (DRUJ) in the setting of a displaced fracture of the base of the ulnar styloid. Subsequently, he also underwent tension-band fixation of this fracture (Fig. 4.2a, b). Therapy focused on early digital, wrist and forearm motion. His post operative hand function was excellent and he was able to return to heavy manual labor (Fig. 4.3a–d).

J.N. Lawton, MD (✉) • J. Hudgens, MD
Department of Orthopaedic Surgery, University of Michigan Health System, A. Alfred Taubman Health Care Center, Floor 2, Reception: B 2912 Taubman Center, 1500 East Medical Center Drive, Ann Arbor, MI 48109-5328, USA
e-mail: jeflawto@med.umich.edu; jhudgens@med.umich.edu

© Springer International Publishing Switzerland 2016   37
J.N. Lawton (ed.), *Distal Radius Fractures*,
DOI 10.1007/978-3-319-27489-8_4

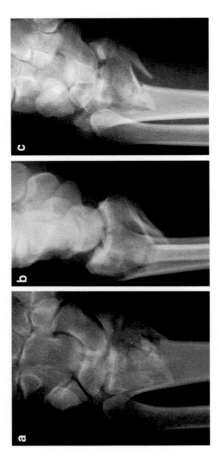

Fig. 4.1 Initial (**a**) anteroposterior (AP), (**b**) lateral, and (**c**) oblique radiographs demonstrating an intra-articular, comminuted distal radius fracture with a substantial radial styloid fragment

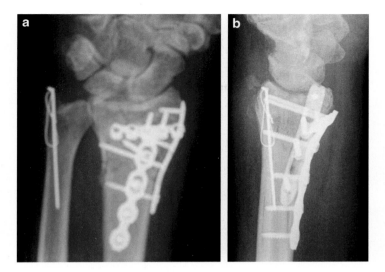

Fig. 4.2 Post operative images, demonstrating fixation of the distal radius with a volar locking plate and radial styloid plate and tension band fixation of the ulnar styloid

Background

The distal radius is one of the most commonly fractured bones [1]. With the primary demographic consisting of young men and elderly women [1], the injury patterns can be quite varied, ranging from simple extra-articular injuries to those with complex articular involvement. Specific fracture patterns may be challenging to manage. AO classification type C2 (complete articular, simple, metaphyseal multifragmentary) and C3 (complete articular, multi-fragmentary) distal radius fractures can include radial column/styloid fragments that can prove difficult to capture with a standard volar locking plate—as the primary or secondary fracture lines would be parallel to the distal screws of most volar plates.

Peine et al. [2] and Rikli and Regazzoni [3] described a three column model of the distal radius and ulna, including a radial column, radial styloid and scaphoid facet, intermediate column, lunate facet and sigmoid notch, and ulnar column, distal ulna and triangular

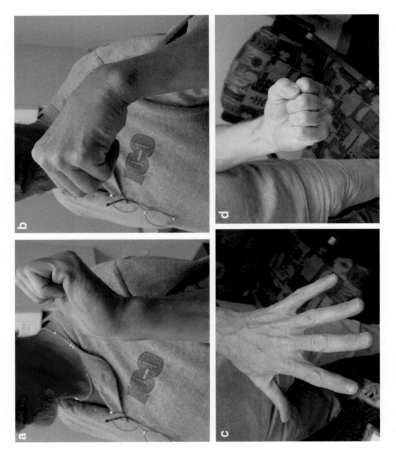

Fig. 4.3 Post operative range of motion

fibrocartilage complex (TFCC). Though the radial styloid only transmits a minor portion of the overall load, as compared the intermediate and ulnar columns, it is critical to the stability of the wrist [4]. Specifically, it functions as an osseous buttress in radial and ulnar deviation, and also forms the origin of the radioscaphocapitate ligament [4].

Fragment-specific fixation, introduced in the late 1990s, advocates the use of low-profile modular implants to fixate specific fracture fragments of the distal radius [5, 6]. Various anatomically designed fragment-specific systems take into account the importance of the radial column and utilize either a radial pin plate or a low-profile plate/screw construct for stabilization of this area, as an integral part of the technique [7]. Dodds et al. [8] examined the fragment-specific system in a biomechanical study that cycled cadaveric wrists through physiologic loads. They noted significantly greater stability, as measured by a 3D motion tracking system, in AO C2 fractures treated with radial and ulnar pin plates as compared to those treated with external fixation alone. Adhering to the concepts of fragment-specific fixation, several have recommended dual plating of the intermediate and radial columns in an orthogonal manner [2, 9, 10]. Peine et al. [2] demonstrated significantly increased stiffness in a cadaveric distal radius fracture model treated with 2.0 mm plates on the radial column and dorsal ulnar surface as compared to dorsal T plate or Pi plate alone (though it should be noted that none of these plates utilized locking technology). Clinical outcome studies of orthogonal plating of the intermediate and radial columns, utilizing fragment-specific implants, have demonstrated good results as well [9, 10]. In addition to dual plating, some have even proposed a benefit of radial plating alone, for a variety of distal radius fracture patterns [11]. A prospective randomized trial comparing locked fixation with either a radial column or volar plate alone demonstrated slightly better patient reported outcomes with a volar plate in the first 3 months. However, both groups had similar clinical results at 6 months, and radial plating actually showed significantly superior maintenance of radial height and inclination at 1 year [11].

Recent Literature

More recently, there has been a trend towards fixation of distal radius fractures through a volar approach, as popularized by Orbay [12], and via a volar locking plate [13]. Despite the mechanical advantages offered by use of these plates, specific fixation of the radial styloid is still important in some fracture patterns. Iba et al. [14] compared matched pairs of cadaveric wrists fixed in an AO C3 type fracture model that were fixed with a locked volar plate with or without two styloid screws. They noted significantly greater ultimate strength to failure in the volar plate group that included styloid screws, underscoring the importance of fixation in this area. Additional biomechanical data has emphasized the importance of styloid fixation particularly with smaller styloid fracture fragments [15]. In a distal AO C3 osteotomy model, Stanbury et al. [15] noted articular failure following load to failure in 8 of 8 specimens plated with a fixed angle volar locking plate, in which the screws follow a pre-determined course. In contrast, none of 8 had articular failure in those stabilized with a variable angle locking plate. They commented that with the variable angle device they were able to place three locking screws into the styloid fragment. However, in a proximal fracture model (with a larger styloid fragment), only 1 of 8 fixed angle and none of 8 variable angle specimens failed.

Despite the utilitarian properties of a locked volar plate, certain fractures may still be better served with a hybrid construct. Grindel et al. [16] compared AO C2 fracture models in cadaveric specimens fixed with either a volar locking plate alone or combined with a radial pin plate. They noted significantly less displacement in distal fragments, during both flexion-extension and radial-ulnar deviation, and also greater stiffness and load to failure in the hybrid group. This method of fixation has been described in the literature by Tang et al. [17] who advocated the use of a radial pin plate in conjunction with a volar locking plate in cases where screw fixation of the styloid fragment may be limited, or in the setting of significantly comminuted intra-articular fractures with a large radial styloid fragment. They also proposed the use of a modified Henry incision, radial to the radial artery, to facilitate radial column exposure. Few studies have directly evaluated the clinical outcomes of this type of hybrid fixation. Jacobi et al. [18] retrospectively reviewed 10 patients with intra-articular distal radius fractures and displacement of the radial styloid. Fractures were fixed with a volar locking plate and either a 2.5 mm or 2.7 mm radial buttress plate. Decision to plate the radial styloid was made intra-operatively if reduction of the styloid fragment was deemed difficult. At 24 months follow-up mean visual analog pain scale (VAS) was 0.9, motion was nearly symmetric to the uninjured side, and good radiographic parameters were noted. However, half of the patients required removal of the radial plate secondary to DeQuervain's type symptoms. Helmerhorst and Kloen [19] also reported the results of 14 patients treated with 2.4 mm locked compression plates for both the volar and radial surfaces of intra-articular distal radius fractures with a concomitant radial column fragment. At 7 weeks, all but one fracture had appeared radiographically healed. No symptoms were noted related to irritation of the first dorsal compartment. At an average of 30-month follow-up, good to excellent functional and radiographic parameters were noted.

Decision Making

A substantial number of distal radius fractures can be stabilized with a volar locking plate alone. We advocate that consideration be given for the addition of radial styloid plate for intra-articular fractures with a separate radial column fragment where a reduction cannot be well maintained with standard methods. Such radial styloid fragments have fracture lines parallel to the traditional screws from volar plate fixation. These scenarios include smaller styloid fragments where it is difficult to place more than 1 locked screw and those fractures with significant comminution and poor bone quality that may benefit from the additional buttressing effect and added rigidity of orthogonal fixation with a radial plate.

Tips and Tricks

1. Consider the radial artery approach based upon pre-operative planning—early identification facilitates an easier dissection.
2. Subperiosteal dissection of brachioradialis allows plate to be protected from 1st dorsal compartment contents.
3. May combine a radial styloid plate with a standard volar plate or with volar ulnar fixation, depending upon fracture pattern.
4. Order of Operations:

   (a) Radial artery approach
   (b) Provisional/definitive radial styloid fixation (often can achieve anatomic reduction)
   (c) K-wire in radial styloid
   (d) Place distal hole of plate over K-wire
   (e) Non-locking transverse screw proximally
   (f) Replace K-wire with locking uni-cortical screw (consider using fluoroscopy to maximize length and minimize risk of joint penetration.)
   (g) Build to the radial styloid with a volar plate

References

1. Court-Brown CM, Caesar B. Epidemiology of adult fractures: a review. Injury. 2006;37(8):691–7.
2. Peine R, Rikli DA, Hoffmann R, Duda G, Regazzoni P. Comparison of three different plating techniques for the dorsum of the distal radius: a biomechanical study. J Hand Surg Am. 2000;25(1):29–33.
3. Rikli DA, Regazzoni P. Fractures of the distal end of the radius treated by internal fixation and early function. A preliminary report of 20 cases. J Bone Joint Surg Br. 1996;78(4):588–92.
4. Rikli DA, Honigmann P, Babst R, Cristalli A, Morlock MM, Mittlmeier T. Intra-articular pressure measurement in the radioulnocarpal joint using a novel sensor: in vitro and in vivo results. J Hand Surg Am. 2007;32(1): 67–75.
5. Medoff RJ, Kopylov P. Immediate internal fixation and motion of comminuted distal radius fractures using a new fragment specific fixation system. Orthop Trans. 1998;22:165.
6. Medoff RJ, Kopylov P. Open reduction and immediate motion of intraarticular distal radius fractures with a fragment specific fixation system. Arch Am Acad Orthop Surg. 1999;2:53–61.

7. Konrath GA, Bahler S. Open reduction and internal fixation of unstable distal radius fractures: results using the trimed fixation system. J Orthop Trauma. 2002;16(8):578–85.

8. Dodds SD, Cornelissen S, Jossan S, Wolfe SW. A biomechanical comparison of fragment-specific fixation and augmented external fixation for intra-articular distal radius fractures. J Hand Surg Am. 2002;27(6):953–64.

9. Chang HC, Poh SY, Seah SC, Chua DT, Cha BK, Low CO. Fragment-specific fracture fixation and double-column plating of unstable distal radial fractures using AO mini-fragment implants and Kirschner wires. Injury. 2007;38(11):1259–67.

10. Jakob M, Rikli DA, Regazzoni P. Fractures of the distal radius treated by internal fixation and early function. A prospective study of 73 consecutive patients. J Bone Joint Surg. 2000;82(3):340–4.

11. Wei DH, Raizman NM, Bottino CJ, Jobin CM, Strauch RJ, Rosenwasser MP. Unstable distal radial fractures treated with external fixation, a radial column plate, or a volar plate. A prospective randomized trial. J Bone Joint Surg Am. 2009;91(7):1568–77.

12. Orbay JL. The treatment of unstable distal radius fractures with volar fixation. Hand Surg. 2000;5(2):103–12.

13. Orbay JL, Fernandez DL. Volar fixed-angle plate fixation for unstable distal radius fractures in the elderly patient. J Hand Surg Am. 2004;29(1): 96–102.

14. Iba K, Ozasa Y, Wada T, Kamiya T, Yamashita T, Aoki M. Efficacy of radial styloid targeting screws in volar plate fixation of intra-articular distal radial fractures: a biomechanical study in a cadaver fracture model. J Orthop Surg Res. 2010;5:90.

15. Stanbury SJ, Salo A, Elfar JC. Biomechanical analysis of a volar variable-angle locking plate: the effect of capturing a distal radial styloid fragment. J Hand Surg Am. 2012;37(12):2488–94.

16. Grindel SI, Wang M, Gerlach M, McGrady LM, Brown S. Biomechanical comparison of fixed-angle volar plate versus fixed-angle volar plate plus fragment-specific fixation in a cadaveric distal radius fracture model. J Hand Surg Am. 2007;32(2):194–9.

17. Tang P, Ding A, Uzumcugil A. Radial column and volar plating (RCVP) for distal radius fractures with a radial styloid component or severe comminution. Tech Hand Up Extrem Surg. 2010;14(3):143–9.

18. Jacobi M, Wahl P, Kohut G. Repositioning and stabilization of the radial styloid process in comminuted fractures of the distal radius using a single approach: the radio-volar double plating technique. J Orthop Surg Res. 2010;5:55.

19. Helmerhorst GT, Kloen P. Orthogonal plating of intra-articular distal radius fractures with an associated radial column fracture via a single volar approach. Injury. 2012;43(8):1307–12.

Chapter 5
Volar Locking Plate for Intra-Articular Distal Radius Fracture

Jennifer Moriatis Wolf

Case Presentation

A 54-year-old college professor presented after a fall on ice with a painful, deformed wrist on her right dominant side. She was evaluated in the emergency department and noted to have mild swelling of the right wrist, with a small volar ulnar superficial abrasion, approximately 2 mm in length, which did not communicate with the deeper tissues. She had intact sensation to light touch in the median, ulnar, and radial nerve distributions.

Radiographs demonstrated a displaced, dorsally angulated, intra-articular distal radius fracture (Fig. 5.1a–c). She underwent closed reduction and sugar tong splint placement in the ED, with improvement in the alignment of the fracture (Fig. 5.2).

She was seen 3 days later in the office with some mild loss of alignment of the right distal radius fracture. Surgical reduction and fixation was recommended due to loss of reduction, with instability of the volar ulnar fragments. She agreed with this recommendation and was brought to the OR the following day.

J.M. Wolf, MD (✉)

Department of Orthopaedic Surgery, University of Connecticut Health Center, 263 Farmington Avenue, Farmington, CT 06030, USA

e-mail: jmwolf@uchc.edu

© Springer International Publishing Switzerland 2016

J.N. Lawton (ed.), *Distal Radius Fractures*,

DOI 10.1007/978-3-319-27489-8_5

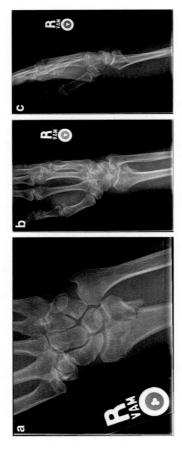

Fig. 5.1 (**a–c**) Posteroanterior, oblique, and lateral radiographs showing a dorsally angulated and displaced distal radius fracture with intra-articular extension and stepoff

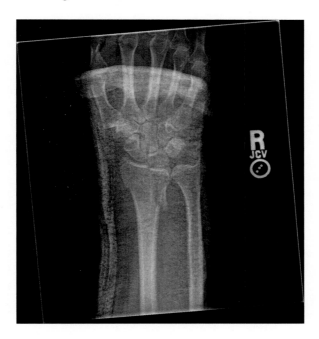

Fig. 5.2 Lateral radiograph showing plaster splint overlying distal radius fracture with improvement in dorsal tilt and partial restoration of radial length, with improvement of the impaction seen on the injury films

Reviewing the fracture, based on what appeared to be a coronal and sagittal split in the distal radial articular surface, we planned a volar approach with plate fixation, with backup plans being a dorsal plate, K-wires, and possible suture fixation of the volar fragments if needed.

We performed a volar approach through the flexor carpi radialis (FCR) tendon sheath (Fig. 5.3), and used 10 lbs of traction across the wrist (hung off the table) to re-align the fragments. We then elevated the fragments using a Freer elevator, and noted a bone gap resulted below the volar lunate fragment due to severe impaction. This was grafted with allograft bone chips, and a volar plate then placed on the fracture, with fixation first placed proximally in the radial shaft to obtain provisional placement. We then fine-tuned

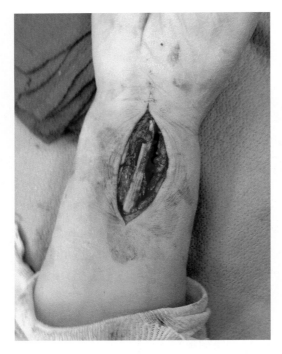

Fig. 5.3 Intra-operative photograph showing volar radial approach to the wrist with exposure of the flexor carpi radialis (FCR) tendon sheath

the position of the plate using fluoroscopic imaging to stay clear of the watershed area and obtain fixation distally, using a combination of locking and non-locking distal screws.

The patient was then placed in a plaster splint and maintained in this for 10 days, and changed to a short arm cast after a wound check and suture removal at that time (Fig. 5.4a–c). She was immobilized for a total of 3 weeks, then transitioned to a short arm thermoplastic splint and started on gentle motion with therapy to optimize motion.

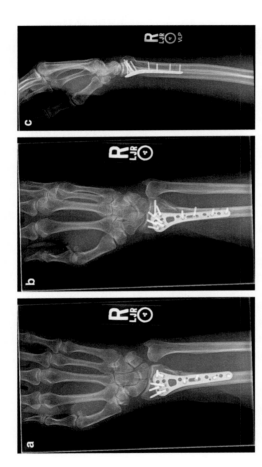

Fig. 5.4 Postoperative posteroanterior, oblique, and lateral radiographs showing volar plate and screw implant transfixing intra-articular distal radius fracture with restoration of length and tilt

Literature Review on the Use of Volar Plate Fixation for Intra-articular Distal Radius Fractures

Volar plating was originally used only for volar Barton's type fractures [1], but the introduction of fixed-angle locking plates, described by Orbay, revolutionized the fixation of distal radius fractures [2]. Other options for surgical fixation include percutaneous Kirschner wires or external fixation. Comparative studies have shown outcomes measures including the Disabilities of the Arm, Shoulder, and Hand scores and motion scores show superiority at 6 and 12 weeks, but measures are essentially equivalent thereafter, up to one year [3–5].

However, two meta-analyses of the literature have indicated that the outcomes of volar plate fixation, in aggregate, are slightly superior to external fixation and other forms of fixation [6, 7], although grip strength outcomes are better with external fixation.

When considering the use of volar plates, it is critical to consider possible complications when using these implants. Complications include flexor tendon rupture or irritation from volar plate prominence [8], extensor tendon rupture or irritation from dorsal screw prominence [9], and intra-articular screw penetration [9]. It is imperative to optimize the technical placement of these plates in order to avoid these complications, with specific attention to not placing the plate too distally, or placing overly long screws.

Choice of Approach: Why and Alternatives

The author chose volar plate fixation for this fracture for two reasons: the open approach that plate fixation allows fragment elevation and bone grafting under the volar ulnar fragment, if needed; and because the plate enables the placement of screws in multiple fragments in a locking fashion to allow a locked construct for stability [10].

Other options would include wire fixation, which would preclude direct fragment visualization and elevation of the depressed volar ulnar fragment and indirect elevation of central fragments (although percutaneous wires or elevators can be used to partially achieve this); external fixation, which would require K-wires to be used to capture the multiple fragments and does not allow wrist motion until after the fixator is removed; or dorsal plating, which would not allow elevation of the volar fragments.

Because of the articular stepoff and the initial dorsal angulation [11] of this fracture, the author would characterize this fracture as unstable and displaced, and thus would not recommend nonoperative treatment as an option.

Tips and Tricks

- Use finger traps, rope, and 10 lb weight hung off the hand table (Fig. 5.5) to provide traction (which often does most of your reduction for you). This is simple and can obviate the need for an assistant.
- Use a Freer elevator to place into the fracture, once under traction, to reduce it. You can palpate the fracture dorsally and palpate the instrument as you pass it along the dorsally angulated fragment so that you know you are at the back to effectively reduce the fracture.
- The author has found it effective to reduce the dorsal fragment first, then to reduce volar fragments up to it. This allows the surgeon to visualize the need for any bone graft, before plate placement.
- Use the lateral view, not the AP, to determine how far distally to place your plate.
- When placing distal screws, if the distal fragments are not badly comminuted, use a non-locking screw first, to draw the fragment up to the plate. This is followed by a locking screw, and then fluoroscopic imaging checked.
- If you open the pronator quadratus with a large radial-sided cuff, it is easier to close over the plate, especially distally.

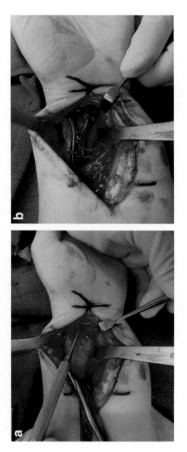

Fig. 5.5 Technique of traction to help with fracture reduction and maintenance of position. Disposable finger traps are attached to sterilized rope, which is hung over the edge of the hand table and can be attached to hanging traction weights. The author typically uses 10 lb of weight, with a rolled towel under the distal fracture fragment to support it and prevent extension

References

1. Axelrod TS, McMurtry RY. Open reduction and internal fixation of comminuted, intraarticular fractures of the distal radius. J Hand Surg Am. 1990;15(1):1–11.
2. Orbay JL. The treatment of unstable distal radius fractures with volar fixation. Hand Surg. 2000;5(2):103–12.
3. Roh YH, Lee BK, Baek JR, Noh JH, Gong HS, Baek GH. A randomized comparison of volar plate and external fixation for intra-articular distal radius fractures. J Hand Surg Am. 2015;40(1):34–41.
4. Williksen JH, Frihagen F, Hellund JC, Kvernmo HD, Husby T. Volar locking plates versus external fixation and adjuvant pin fixation in unstable distal radius fractures: a randomized, controlled study. J Hand Surg Am. 2013;38(8):1469–76.
5. Wright TW, Horodyski M, Smith DW. Functional outcome of unstable distal radius fractures: ORIF with a volar fixed-angle tine plate versus external fixation. J Hand Surg Am. 2005;30(2):289–99.
6. Wei DH, Poolman RW, Bhandari M, Wolfe VM, Rosenwasser MP. External fixation versus internal fixation for unstable distal radius fractures: a systematic review and meta-analysis of comparative clinical trials. J Orthop Trauma. 2012;26(7):386–94.
7. Esposito J, Schemitsch EH, Saccone M, Sternheim A, Kuzyk PR. External fixation versus open reduction with plate fixation for distal radius fractures: a meta-analysis of randomised controlled trials. Injury. 2013;44(4): 409–16.
8. Kitay A, Swanstrom M, Schreiber JJ, Carlson MG, Nguyen JT, Weiland AJ, Daluiski A. Volar plate position and flexor tendon rupture following distal radius fracture fixation. J Hand Surg Am. 2013;38(6):1091–6.
9. Tarallo L, Mugnai R, Zambianchi F, Adani R, Catani F. Volar plate fixation for the treatment of distal radius fractures: analysis of adverse events. J Orthop Trauma. 2013;27(12):740–5.
10. Orbay JL, Touhami A. Current concepts in volar fixed-angle fixation of unstable distal radius fractures. Clin Orthop Relat Res. 2006;445:58–67.
11. Leung F, Ozkan M, Chow SP. Conservative treatment of intra-articular fractures of the distal radius–factors affecting functional outcome. Hand Surg. 2000;5(2):145–53.

Chapter 6
Dorsal Plate Fixation for Distal Radius Fractures

J.M. Kirsch, E.P. Tannenbaum, and J.N. Lawton

Case Presentation

A 60-year-old right-hand-dominant female with osteoporosis presented to our Emergency Department following a fall from a 10-foot tall ladder onto her outstretched right hand while she was painting her ceiling. Her clinical examination demonstrated an obvious deformity at the wrist with diffuse swelling and tenderness to palpation over the distal radius. Her neurovascular examination was unremarkable.

PA and lateral plain radiographs of her right wrist demonstrated a dorsally displaced, intra-articular distal radius fracture (Figs. 6.1 and 6.2). A closed reduction was successfully performed under a local hematoma block and the patient was placed in a sugar tong splint. At her follow-up clinic visit, repeat radiographs demonstrated loss of her volar tilt with approximately 12 degrees of dorsal angulation (Figs. 6.3 and 6.4). Based upon her initial displacement,

J.M. Kirsch, MD (✉) • E.P. Tannenbaum, MD • J.N. Lawton, MD
Department of Orthopaedic Surgery, University of Michigan Health
System, A. Alfred Taubman Health Care Center, Floor 2, Reception: B,
2912 Taubman Center, 1500 East Medical Center Drive,
Ann Arbor, MI 48109-5328, USA
e-mail: kirschj@med.umich.edu; erictann@med.umich.edu;
jeflawto@med.umich.edu

© Springer International Publishing Switzerland 2016   57
J.N. Lawton (ed.), *Distal Radius Fractures*,
DOI 10.1007/978-3-319-27489-8_6

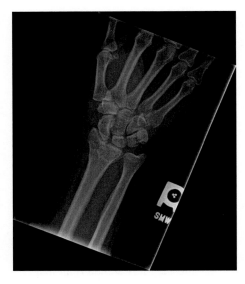

Fig. 6.1 Injury PA demonstrating apparent loss of radial length which is, in reality, just dorsal angulation as appreciated better on the lateral projection

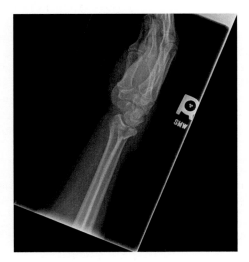

Fig. 6.2 Injury lateral demonstrating dorsal angulation with intra-articular comminution. Note the greater impaction and displacement dorsally with the relatively simpler pattern volarly

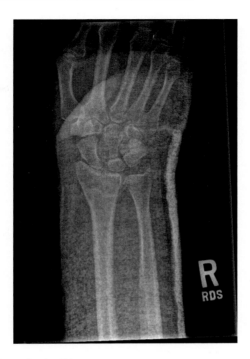

Fig. 6.3 Post-reduction PA

residual displacement, intra-articular involvement, and her activity level, the decision was made to perform open reduction and internal fixation to improve her alignment.

Given the fracture pattern involving a comminuted dorsal wall fracture fragment, a dorsal approach was chosen with the use of dorsal plating. An incision was made over Lister's tubercle dissecting down through the subcutaneous tissue to the third dorsal compartment, which was incised while being mindful of the Extensor Pollicis Longus (EPL) tendon. Next, a subperiosteal approach was performed under the 2nd and 4th dorsal compartments and the fracture fragments were reduced. Comminution of the radial styloid and lunate facet was also noted. An Acumed (Hillsboro, OR) dorsal distal radius plate was then secured first proximally with non-locking screws and then distally with locking screws. Appropriate fracture reduction and hardware placement

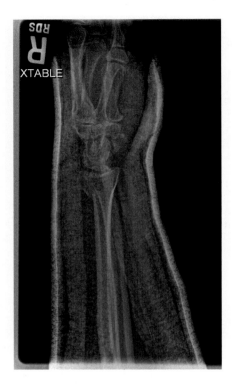

Fig. 6.4 Post-reduction lateral x-ray demonstrating improved alignment, however the lunate appears to be translatted slightly dorsally with the dorsal articular fragment

was subsequently confirmed using intraoperative fluoroscopy and the wound was irrigated and closed in a layered fashion with the EPL left subcutaneously. Finally, the patient was placed into a well-padded above-the-elbow splint with her arm supinated.

At her initial 2-week post-operative clinic visit, the patient was doing well. Her post-operative radiographs can be seen in Figs. 6.5 and 6.6. She was transitioned into an orthoplast clamshell splint and instructed to begin working on range of motion exercises for her wrist. She reported that she had returned to all of her normal activities at her 10-week clinic visit (Fig. 6.7).

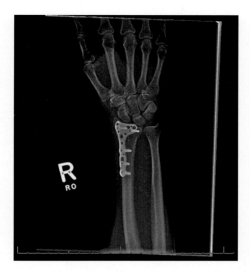

Fig. 6.5 Post-Op PA

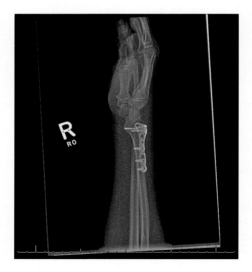

Fig. 6.6 Post-Op lateral

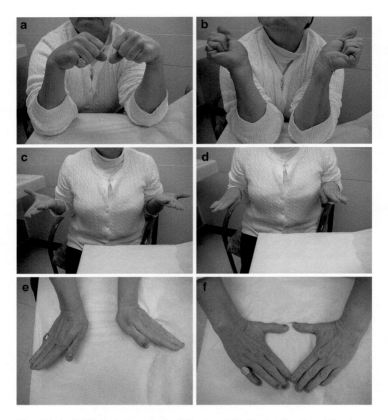

Fig. 6.7 (**a–f**) Clinical photographs following right distal radius dorsal fixation

Background

A paradigm shift in the surgical treatment of distal radius fractures has occurred over the course of the past decade, currently favoring plate fixation. A Swedish study in 2013 noted that the use of plate fixation for treating distal radius increased by more than 400 % over a 6-year period [1]. Furthermore, the preferred method of plate fixation has also changed. Dorsal plates were commonly used in the 1980s for dorsally displaced and dorsally angulated fractures. Advocates of this technique favored the ability to have direct visualization of the articular surface and believed there was a biomechanical advantage to having a dorsal buttress for dorsally angulated fractures. However, today is it commonplace for these fractures to be treated through a volar approach and only rarely is a dorsal approach considered.

Dorsal plating has fallen out of favor primarily due to high rates of extensor tendon complications; most of which occurred using traditional 2.5 mm thick plates. Patients treated with volar plates did not have as many complications; therefore, this approach became more favorable. Although, newer reports demonstrate that extensor tendon complications are possible following volar plating as well [2]. New dorsal plates were subsequently designed to address the complications seen in their predecessors. These plates come in a variety of pre-contoured sizes with a 1.2–1.5 mm thick low-profile design and rounded, tapered edges to help minimize extensor tendon irritation. Additionally, low-profile dorsal plates are available with fixed and variable angle locking screw heads that are flush to the plate. This design attempts to avoid potential extensor tendon complications while allowing for optimal fixation in poor quality bone. Despite the modifications with newer generation dorsal plates, volar plating remains the more popular option for treating distal radius fractures.

Current literature demonstrates that low-profile dorsal plates have substantially fewer complications compared to traditional high-profile plates. Most of this difference is due to the nearly 50 % reduction in plate thickness. Rozental and colleagues compared the functional outcomes and complications in patients treated with traditional dorsal plates to those treated with low-profile plates. Nearly half of the patients treated with traditional plates had complications requiring surgical removal of the plate or extensor tendon reconstruction, whereas none of the patients in their study who were treated with a low-profile plate required this intervention [3]. Furthermore, they reported excellent long-term functional outcomes with the low-profile plates. Rein and colleagues also reported a similar 50 % complication rate with traditional 2.5 mm dorsal plates [4]. Kamath et al. reported excellent functional outcomes in 93 % of patients treated with a low-profile dorsal plate at an average of 18 months of follow-up. Additionally, 70 % of the patients in their study had highly comminuted intra-articular fractures, and none of them demonstrated fracture displacement or required plate removal [5]. Another study looking at 51 distal radius fractures treated with a low-profile dorsal plates reported zero cases of extensor tendon complications, nonunions, infections, or nerve injuries at 2 years of follow-up [6].

Low-profile dorsal plates have also compared very favorably to volar plates in treating distal radius fractures. A recent large meta-analysis comparing low-profile dorsal plates and volar plates in over 950 patients demonstrated no significant difference in the overall complication rate, risk of tendon rupture, frequency of screw loosening, or risk of developing complex regional pain syndrome (CRPS). Furthermore, the authors found a significantly higher risk of neuropathy and carpal tunnel syndrome with volar plating [7]. Yu and colleagues reported similar results, demonstrating no significant difference between low-profile dorsal plates and volar plates regarding rates of tendon irritation or rupture, hardware discomfort, infection, or CRPS. They too found a significantly higher incidence of neuropathy with volar plating. Additionally, all of their patients with neuropathy required additional surgical intervention [8]. Recent biomechanical data has produced mixed results, with some authors demonstrating no difference between dorsal and volar plates [9], whereas some studies indicate a biomechanical advantage to dorsal plating [10].

Advantages

The unique advantages of dorsal plating for distal radius fractures include: the opportunity for the surgeon to visualize the articular surface to help ensure an anatomic reduction, particularly with depressed and highly comminuted intra-articular fragments; being able to adequately visualize and address the extent of dorsal comminution common in fractures with osteoporotic bone; the ability to evaluate and intervene in cases of intercarpal ligamentous injury and obtaining better fixation in specific fracture types.

Achieving an anatomic reduction is always ideal to give the patient the best opportunity to have an excellent functional outcome and prevent posttraumatic arthrosis. This can be sometimes difficult through a volar approach, particularly in patients with poor bone quality who sustain complex intra-articular depression fractures. A dorsal approach allows for the best visualization of the distal radial articular surface and the dorsal surface, which is often comminuted with areas of bony deficiency. In cases of dorsal bone defects, it is possible to use allograft bone chips or iliac crest bone graft to provide structural support. Additionally, Wichlas and colleagues found that dorsal plating was better able to reestablish adequate volar tilt and ulnar variance compared to the volar plates [11].

Lutsky and colleagues recognized the ability to assess for intercarpal ligamentous injury at the time of distal radius fixation as a key advantage to dorsal plating, since both can be repaired using the same dorsal approach [12]. In particular, scapholunate interosseous ligament (SLIL) injury is often overlooked when treating distal radius fractures. One can evaluate the integrity of the SLIL intraoperatively either by arthroscopy or by direct visualization after a capsulotomy of the radiocarpal joint. The reported incidence of SLIL injury with a concomitant distal radius fracture varies in the literature. In one study, Richards et al. noted that 22 % of intra-articular fractures had SLIL injury, whereas it was present in only 7 % of extra-articular fractures [13]. In another study, Mehta et al. reported that 85 % of intra-articular distal radius fractures were found to have SLIL injury during arthroscopy [14]. Forward and colleagues noted that patients with intra-articular fractures had a twofold increased risk of scapholunate dissociation by 1 year. Additionally, increased ulnar variance of >2 mm on the injured side was associated with a fourfold increased risk of having a grade 3 SLIL injury [15]. Recent data has also reaffirmed that acute surgical intervention for SLIL injuries produces superior outcomes with less failure rates [16]. Early recognition and intervention is important because the natural history of SLIL injury is believed to be one of progressive global carpal dysfunction ultimately culminating in scapholunate advanced collapse (SLAC) arthritis in some individuals. However, some authors question the predictability of this outcome [17].

In a recent review article, Lutsky also highlighted specific fracture types in which dorsal plating is the preferred surgical technique [12]. Dorsal Barton's or dorsal shear type fractures result from a fall on an outstretched extended wrist causing the carpus to fracture the dorsal radial articular rim. The articular fracture fragment displaces dorsally and proximally and the carpus will often dislocate with it. These fractures are often not amenable to closed reduction as the fragment is unstable and will displace. Additionally, a die-punch fracture is a depression fracture of the lunate fossa resulting from the lunate compressing into the articular surface of the radius. This usually results in a dorsally displaced articular fragment, however the carpus is stable, unlike in the dorsal Barton's fracture. Both of these fracture patterns typically result in a dorsally displaced articular fragment and would benefit from dorsal buttressing. Utilizing a dorsal approach for these fractures results in exceptional exposure of the fracture fragments and the articular surface. Additionally, it provides an opportunity to augment the fixation with bone graft.

Indications

The optimal treatment strategy for distal radius fractures remains an area of controversy. Patients with unstable fracture patterns, or with fractures that fail to maintain an acceptable reduction with closed techniques often require operative intervention. According to the most recent recommendations from the American Academy of Orthopaedic Surgeons, surgical fixation is indicated when there is post-reduction radial shortening >3 mm, dorsal tilt >10°, or intra-articular displacement or step-off >2 mm [18]. There are several specific fracture patterns in which a dorsal exposure with a dorsally placed plate is more advantageous compared to a volar approach. As a general principle, highly comminuted intra-articular fractures that are dorsally displaced with dorsal bony deficiency or comminution in patients with osteoporotic bone or in cases of a high-energy mechanism are ideal candidates for considering a dorsal approach with a low-profile dorsal plate. The ability to obtain a good articular exposure also allows for optimal reduction of depressed intra-articular fragments. Dorsal plating has been used successfully in a wide variety of distal radius fractures including AO type A (extra-articular fractures), AO type B (partial articular shear fractures), and all subtypes of AO type C (complete articular fractures), which can have high degrees of intra-articular and metaphyseal comminution [19].

Contraindications

Generally speaking, it is inadvisable to operate and implant hardware in patients who are poor surgical candidates or have grossly infected tissues. While some studies have indicated that individuals older than 55 years can have good outcomes with nonsurgical treatment, most surgeons consider open reduction and internal fixation for displaced fractures in active patients [18]. Additionally, dorsal plating is not advisable when the dominant fragment is volarly displaced or angulated, such as in cases of volar Barton's or volar shear fractures. In cases when the volar fragment is substantially larger than the dorsal fragment, some authors have found that dorsally placed screws may not sufficiently capture the volar fragment, predisposing to potential collapse [19]. Additionally, in highly comminuted fractures, one must be careful not to over-reduce the fracture and volarly translate the distal radius and the carpus.

Tips/Tricks

- Repeating fluoroscopy with stress views may reveal a more complex fracture pattern than was initially appreciated with the hand at rest.
- It is imperative to look for and identify the superficial branch of the radial nerve (SBRN) during the surgical approach. It can usually be found just deep to the subcutaneous tissue, 7–9 cm proximal to the tip of the radial styloid. One of the terminal branches

can often be observed crossing the extensor pollicis longus (EPL) tendon heading in an ulnar and dorsal direction [12].

- A careful subperiosteal dissection of the dorsal compartments will allow the periosteum to act as a protective layer between the plate and the extensor tendons.
- A brachioradialis release may help facilitate fracture reduction and minimize it as a deforming force upon the styloid fragment.
- Some authors have estimated that in approximately 2 % of cases of highly comminuted fractures, the EPL tendon can become trapped in-between fracture fragments. In these instances, it is essential to recognize this early, because further traction on the hand in an attempt to reduce the fracture will only pull the tendon further in-between fracture fragments making reduction impossible. This also highlights another advantage to the dorsal approach, since visualization of the entrapped tendon would have been impossible if approached volarly [19].
- Bicortical screw purchase is not necessary when using locking plates for distal radius fractures. Adequate stability can be achieved with screws measuring 75 % of the anterior–posterior cortical distance [20].
- Early ROM, afforded by a stable construct, following surgery with a subsequent formal therapy program helps improve functional outcomes.

References

1. Wilcke MKT, Hammarberg H, Adolphson PY. Epidemiology and changed surgical treatment methods for fractures of the distal radius: a registry analysis of 42,583 patients in Stockholm County, Sweden, 2004–2010. Acta Orthop. 2013;84(3):292–6. doi:10.3109/17453674.2013.792035.
2. Arora R, Lutz M, Hennerbichler A, Krappinger D, Espen D, Gabl M. Complications following internal fixation of unstable distal radius fracture with a palmar locking-plate. J Orthop Trauma. 2007;21(5):316–22. doi:10.1097/BOT.0b013e318059b993.
3. Rozental TD, Beredjiklian PK, Bozentka DJ. Functional outcome and complications following two types of dorsal plating for unstable fractures of the distal part of the radius. J Bone Joint Surg. 2003;85-A(10):1956–60.

4. Rein S, Schikore H, Schneiders W, Amlang M, Zwipp H. Results of dorsal or volar plate fixation of AO type C3 distal radius fractures: a retrospective study. J Hand Surg Am. 2007;32(7):954–61. doi:10.1016/j.jhsa.2007.05.008.

5. Kamath AF, Zurakowski D, Day CS. Low-profile dorsal plating for dorsally angulated distal radius fractures: an outcomes study. J Hand Surg Am. 2006;31(7):1061–7. doi:10.1016/j.jhsa.2006.05.008.

6. Simic PM, Robison J, Gardner MJ, Gelberman RH, Weiland AJ, Boyer MI. Treatment of distal radius fractures with a low-profile dorsal plating system: an outcomes assessment. J Hand Surg Am. 2006;31(3):382–6. doi:10.1016/j.jhsa.2005.10.016.

7. Wei J, Yang T-B, Luo W, Qin J-B, Kong F-J. Complications following dorsal versus volar plate fixation of distal radius fracture: a meta-analysis. J Int Med Res. 2013;41(2):265–75. doi:10.1177/0300060513476438.

8. Yu YR, Makhni MC, Tabrizi S, Rozental TD, Mundanthanam G, Day CS. Complications of low-profile dorsal versus volar locking plates in the distal radius: a comparative study. J Hand Surg Am. 2011;36(7):1135–41. doi:10.1016/j.jhsa.2011.04.004.

9. McCall TA, Conrad B, Badman B, Wright T. Volar versus dorsal fixed-angle fixation of dorsally unstable extra-articular distal radius fractures: a biomechanic study. J Hand Surg Am. 2007;32(6):806–12. doi:10.1016/j.jhsa.2007.04.016.

10. Blythe M, Stoffel K, Jarrett P, Kuster M. Volar versus dorsal locking plates with and without radial styloid locking plates for the fixation of dorsally comminuted distal radius fractures: a biomechanical study in cadavers. J Hand Surg Am. 2006;31(10):1587–93. doi:10.1016/j.jhsa.2006.09.011.

11. Wichlas F, Haas NP, Disch A, Machó D, Tsitsilonis S. Complication rates and reduction potential of palmar versus dorsal locking plate osteosynthesis for the treatment of distal radius fractures. J Orthop Traumatol. 2014. doi:10.1007/s10195-014-0306-y.

12. Lutsky K, Boyer M, Goldfarb C. Dorsal locked plate fixation of distal radius fractures. J Hand Surg Am. 2013;38(7):1414–22. doi:10.1016/j.jhsa.2013.04.019.

13. Richards RS, Bennett JD, Roth JH, Milne K. Arthroscopic diagnosis of intra-articular soft tissue injuries associated with distal radial fractures. J Hand Surg Am. 1997;22(5):772–6. doi:10.1016/S0363-5023(97)80068-8.

14. Mehta JA, Bain GI, Heptinstall RJ. Anatomical reduction of intra-articular fractures of the distal radius. An arthroscopically-assisted approach. J Bone Joint Surg Br. 2000;82(1):79–86.

15. Forward DP, Lindau TR, Melsom DS. Intercarpal ligament injuries associated with fractures of the distal part of the radius. J Bone Joint Surg. 2007. doi:10.1016/S0021-9355(07)73206-X.

16. Rohman EM, Agel J, Putnam MD, Adams JE. Scapholunate interosseous ligament injuries: a retrospective review of treatment and outcomes in 82 wrists. J Hand Surg Am. 2014;39(10):2020–6. doi:10.1016/j.jhsa.2014.06.139.

17. Strauch RJ. Scapholunate advanced collapse and scaphoid nonunion advanced collapse arthritis—update on evaluation and treatment. J Hand Surg Am. 2011;36(4):729–35. doi:10.1016/j.jhsa.2011.01.018.

18. Lichtman DM, Bindra RR, Boyer MI, et al. Treatment of distal radius fractures. J Am Acad Orthop Surg. 2010;18(3):180–9.

19. Carneiro RS, Radi-Peters C, Goncalves R. Dorsal plate fixation. In: Slutsky D, Osterman L, editors. Fractures and injuries of the distal radius and carpus. Philadelphia, Saunders; 2009. p. 117–123.

20. Wall LB, Brodt MD, Silva MJ, Boyer MI, Calfee RP. The effects of screw length on stability of simulated osteoporotic distal radius fractures fixed with volar locking plates. J Hand Surg Am. 2012;37(3):446–53. doi:10.1016/j.jhsa.2011.12.013.

Chapter 7
Fragment-Specific Internal Fixation of Distal Radius Fractures

Ryan A. Mlynarek and Jeffrey N. Lawton

Case History

A 22-year-old right-hand dominant woman sustained a fall on an outstretched left hand while rollerblading. She experienced immediate pain in the left wrist and presented to the emergency department. Posteroanterior (PA), lateral, and oblique radiographs of the left wrist were obtained (Fig. 7.1), revealing a comminuted intra-articular distal radius fracture, with involvement of the radial column, dorsal wall, and dorsal-ulnar corner. There was also an associated ulnar styloid avulsion. She denied any previous trauma to the wrist and was otherwise healthy. Her wrist was splinted and she presented to clinic for further evaluation of her injury.

The risks and benefits of nonoperative and operative management were discussed with the patient. Given the fracture pattern, we discussed operative treatment using fragment-specific fixation techniques with the patient—including the need for a second operation to remove the dorsal hardware once union was achieved. Given the severity of the fracture with intra-articular extension, as well as the patient's desire to return to her previous activity level

R.A. Mlynarek, MD (✉) • J.N. Lawton, MD
Department of Orthopaedic Surgery, University of Michigan Health System, A. Alfred Taubman Health Care Center, Floor 2, Reception: B, 2912 Taubman Center, 1500 East Medical Center Drive, Ann Arbor, MI 48109-5328, USA
e-mail: mlynarek@med.umich.edu

© Springer International Publishing Switzerland 2016   71
J.N. Lawton (ed.), *Distal Radius Fractures*,
DOI 10.1007/978-3-319-27489-8_7

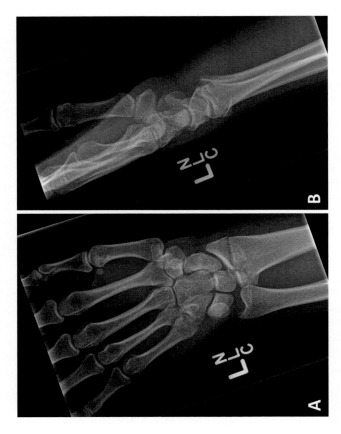

Fig. 7.1 Posteroanterior (PA) and lateral radiographs of the left wrist, revealing a comminuted intra-articular distal radius fracture with large radial styloid and dorsal-ulnar corner fragments

without significant limitation or pain, the patient elected to undergo open reduction and internal fixation of her distal radius.

The patient was taken to the operating room 4 days after her injury. Given the nature of the fracture, we elected to treat this injury using fragment-specific plating with utilization of two incisions. The radial aspect of distal radius was approached over the radial artery with dissection through the subcutaneous tissues to protect branches of the superficial radial sensory nerve. The Brachioradialis was incised sub-periosteally, representing the floor of the first dorsal compartment; and the abductor pollicis longus (APL) and extensor pollicis brevis (EPB) tendons were retracted dorsally (Fig. 7.2). Release of the Brachioradialis insertion off the radial styloid limits its deforming force to allow for adequate fragment mobilization and

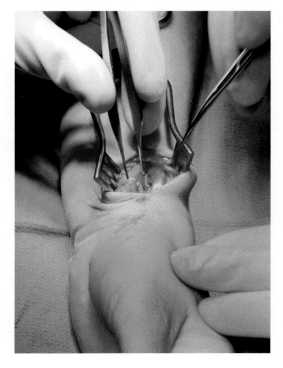

Fig. 7.2 The first dorsal compartment is incised along the Brachioradialis insertion deep to the Abductor Pollicis Longus (APL) and Extensor Pollicis Brevis (EPB) tendons which were retracted dorsally

reduction (Fig. 7.3a). The fragment was then reduced and provisionally stabilized using a single Kirschner wire (Fig. 7.3b). A radial
styloid fragment-specific plate was then secured to the diaphysis
with non-locking cortical screws. As a technical tip, this provisional
K-wire is placed through a hole in the Radial Styloid Plate and later
exchanged for a locking unicortical screw. Flexion and extension of
the wrist was performed under fluoroscopy, as the lunate exhibited
dorsal subluxation/escape with the dorsal-ulnar corner fragment—

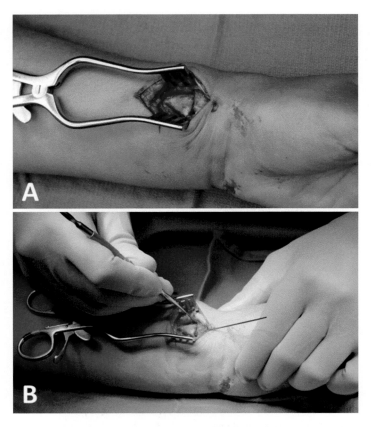

Fig. 7.3 (**a**) The Brachioradialis insertion is sub-periosteally elevated to limit
the deforming force to allow for fragment mobilization and reduction using a
single K-wire (**b**)

demonstrating its critical importance to rigidly internally fix (Fig. 7.4) (for further discussion see Chap. 3).

We then turned our attention to the dorsal-ulnar aspect of the wrist, where a longitudinal incision was made over the third dorsal compartment (Fig. 7.5). The EPL tendon was then mobilized radially, and the floor of the third dorsal compartment was incised, allowing for a sub-periosteal approach to the dorsal wrist under the fourth dorsal compartment. The dorsal-ulnar corner was reduced and an L-shaped fragment-specific stainless steel plate was provisionally placed. The plate was under-contoured to allow for a spring-plate type effect, and the fragment was reduced anatomically and secured to the diaphysis with non-locking cortical screws (Fig. 7.6).

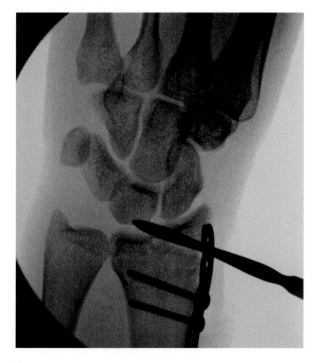

Fig. 7.4 The wrist is flexed and extended under fluoroscopy, demonstrating dorsal subluxation/escape of the lunate secondary to instability of the dorsal-ulnar corner fragment

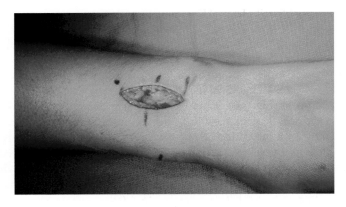

Fig. 7.5 A dorsal incision is made over the third dorsal extensor compartment

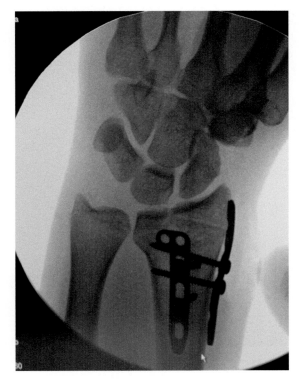

Fig. 7.6 Interval placement of an under-contoured ʟ-shaped fragment-specific stainless steel plate to reduce the dorsal-ulnar corner fragment and allow for a spring-plate type effect

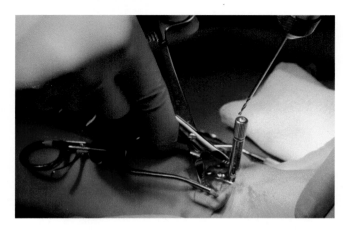

Fig. 7.7 The radial styloid fracture fragment is reduced and compressed using a lobster claw clamp, and a locking peri-articular screw was placed

Attention was then brought back to the radial styloid fragment. Reduction and compression of the fracture were achieved by utilizing a lobster claw clamp, and a single locking peri-articular screw was placed (Fig. 7.7). The articular surface was then reevaluated to confirm anatomic reduction, the wrist was manipulated to ensure stability of the distal radial ulnar joint, and final fluoroscopic images were obtained (Fig. 7.8). The subcutaneous tissue and skin were then closed in layers after tourniquet deflation and hemostasis was achieved, and the patient was placed into a sugartong splint in supination.

The patient was then seen in clinic 2 weeks postoperatively, where her splint and sutures were removed and she began a supervised therapy program of digital/wrist/forearm ROM. The patient was then seen in clinic at 6 weeks, 10 weeks, and 6 months postoperatively (Figs. 7.9 and 7.10). The patient's range of motion in flexion, extension, supination and pronation was identical to the contralateral side. At 9 months postoperatively, she underwent elective removal of hardware.

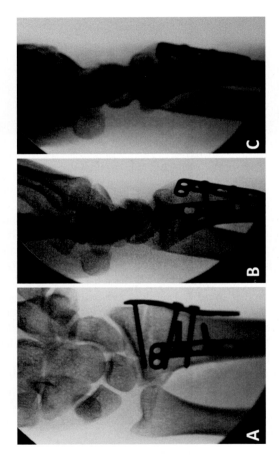

Fig. 7.8 Final PA (**a**), lateral (**b**), and oblique (**c**) fluoroscopic views taken intra-operatively to confirm anatomic reduction

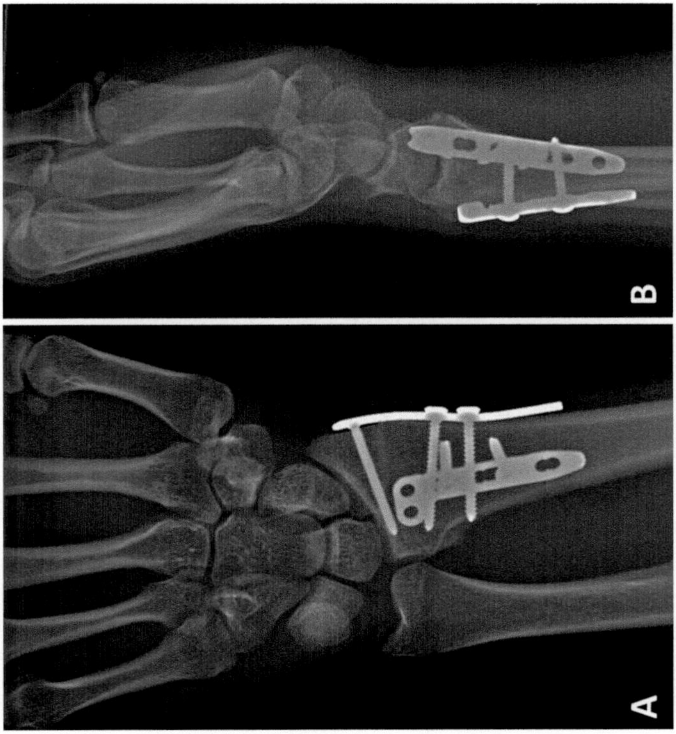

Fig. 7.9 PA (**a**) and lateral (**b**) radiographs of the left wrist at 6-weeks follow-up, revealing maintenance of reduction and interval healing of fracture with minimal callus formation

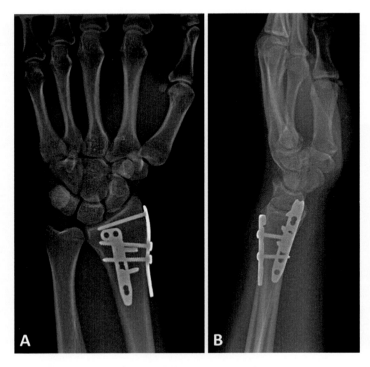

Fig. 7.10 PA (**a**) and lateral (**b**) radiographs of the left wrist at 6-month follow-up, revealing anatomic reduction of previous fracture

Background Information

The distal radius is the most common location of fracture experienced in the upper extremity, with 50 % involving the articular surface [1, 2]. These injuries have long been known to cause significant pain and disability if left untreated [3–7]. In fact, it has been shown that articular malreduction of 1–2 mm can lead to posttraumatic radiographic radiocarpal arthritis in 90 % of patients at an average of 6.7 years follow-up, as well as pain and stiffness at an average of 38-month follow-up [8, 9]. Thus, numerous methods of fixation have been developed to treat these fractures and minimize radiocarpal and radioulnar incongruity. Volar and dorsal plating systems are designed to capture most fragments to a single plate and achieve rigid fixation. Dorsal plating alone has fallen out of favor recently secondary to complications of attritional tendon irritation, rupture, and loss of fracture reduction [10, 11]. However, studies have shown that low-profile dorsal plating with anatomic pre-contoured implants may not be associated with as high of rates of extensor tendon injury as previously described [12, 13]. The advent of volar plate fixation has enabled surgeons to achieve anatomic reduction in the great majority of these fractures, while eluding many of the complications associated with dorsal plating [10, 11, 14–16]. Although this approach may be adequate for the majority of simple fracture patterns, fragment-specific fixation was developed to address complex distal radius fractures that were previously challenging to treat with single-plate fixation [17, 18]. Fragment-specific fixation is performed by addressing all fracture fragments independently with small plates, pins, or wire-forms to anatomically reduce the fracture with adequate biomechanical stability to enable early rehabilitation. This technique has the additional advantage of smaller implants/dissection which may be more friendly to soft tissues during the patient's rehabilitation [19].

Surgical Technique

Multiple classification systems have been developed to describe distal radius fractures, as described in the previous chapters [4, 20–22]. An intra-articular fragment-specific classification was developed by Leslie and Medoff in 2000, which describes the five major fragments (Fig. 7.11) [23]. These include the radial styloid, the dorsal wall, the dorsal-ulnar corner, the volar rim, and impacted articular fragments. The basis of fragment-specific fixation hinges upon one's ability to identify each of these major fragments present and address them individually to create a stable anatomic reduction.

Two to three incisions are routinely used to gain adequate articular reduction. The distal volar Henry approach can be used to

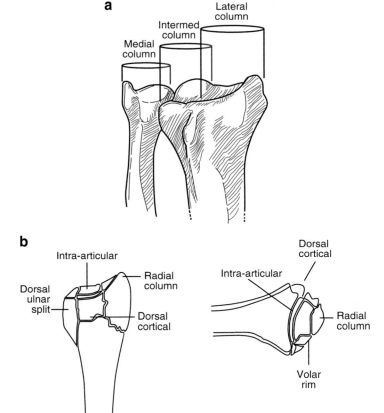

Fig. 7.11 (**a**) The three-column concept of the articular surface of the wrist and the fragment-specific classification (**b**)

address volar rim, radial column, and impacted articular fragments. This approach is made between the ulnar border of the radial artery and the radial border of the flexor carpi radialis (FCR). FCR is then retracted ulnarly and an incision is made through the FCR subsheath. Flexor pollicis longus (FPL) is then retracted ulnarly and Pronator Quadratus (PQ) is elevated and mobilized ulnarly to access the volar radius. A more direct radial approach may be utilized as described above to address radial styloid fragments without volar comminution—absent a need to access the scaphoid/lunate facets. A dorsal incision, also described in our case example, may be used to effectively treat fractures involving the dorsal wall, dorsal-ulnar corner, and impacted articular fragments. Generally, dorsal comminution is addressed first and provisional stabilization is utilized in an ulnar-to-radial direction [24]. Traction is utilized to reestablish length, and ligamentotaxis assists with fracture reduction. A capsulotomy may be performed to remove intra-articular soft tissue or debris which may block reduction. A combination of small contoured low-profile plates and wire-forms can be used to gain anatomic reduction with orthogonal fixation.

Outcomes

In recent years, there has been an increasing number of biomechanical stability and clinical outcome data studies reported using fragment-specific fixation. In 2002, Dodds et al. showed that fragment-specific fixation provided greater stability in comminuted fractures when compared to augmented external fixation [25]. Harness et al. reported that the stability of complex intra-articular fractures depends on the reduction and fixation of smaller fragments, specifically the volar lunate fragment, which can easily be achieved with fragment-specific fixation [26]. With this biomechanical advantage, patients are able to begin a program of early active mobilization, which has been shown to result in good to excellent clinical outcomes [27]. When compared to fixed-angle volar plating, Taylor et al. found that fragment-specific fixation of type C2 fractures revealed no significant difference in cyclical load to failure, however did have improved stiffness characteristics with respect to the ulnar-sided fragments [28]. Similarly, Cooper et al. in 2007 found no significant difference in stiffness when comparing volar locking-screw plating versus fragment-specific fixation in extra-articular cadaveric distal radius fractures with dorsal comminution, but found significantly less linear displacement and mean angulation after osteotomy when using fragment-specific fixation [29]. Their findings indicate that fragment-specific fixation provides significantly more stability than volar locking plates at load magnitudes expected during postoperative rehabilitation.

In 2006, Benson et al. reported clinical outcomes of 85 intra-articular distal radius fractures (AO types: 31 C1, 27 C2, and 18 C3) treated with fragment-specific fixation with a mean follow-up of 32 months [30]. They reported good to excellent results with respect to range of motion, grip strength, radiographic alignment, and satisfaction scoring. Likewise, Gavaskar et al. reported a prospective trial of 105 consecutive patients over 24 months (AO types: 41 C1, 31 C2, and 33 C3) who were treated with fragment-specific fixation [31]. They found 96 % of patients returned to their original occupation at a mean of 58 days, with significant improvements in DASH and PRWE clinical outcome scoring. Konrath et al. has reported on 27 patients treated with fragment-specific fixation with 2-year follow-up, finding high patient satisfaction scores, as well as excellent clinical and radiographic outcomes, with only 1 patient who had experienced loss of fracture reduction requiring reoperation [18].

Complications

There is often significant soft tissue damage associated with complex intra-articular distal radius fractures, which can result in marked swelling. In most cases, two incisions will be utilized to achieve reduction using fragment-specific fixation, and therefore surgical timing and soft tissue management are exceedingly important. Nerve and tendon injuries are not uncommonly associated with these fractures and should be thoroughly assessed prior to definitive bony fixation [32]. Properly placed and secured pins minimize the risk of hardware loosening, but pin migration may cause crepitus, pain, and soft tissue irritation. One must be meticulous about K-wire length and ensure engagement of the cortical bone to minimize loosening. Tendon irritation or rupture may be a concern when using the fragment-specific fixation technique;

however, significant improvements in creating low-profile pre-contoured plates, pins, and wire-forms have decreased this risk substantially [12, 13]. Benson et al. reported that hardware removal was required in 5/85 (5.8 %) wrists after fragment-specific fixation secondary to pain in the area of either a radial styloid or dorsal plate, which was resolved after hardware removal [30]. When direct radial and dorsal fixation is utilized as in our patient's case above, it is our preference to offer hardware removal to those patients if symptomatic.

Considering the osteoporotic population in which distal radius fractures most commonly occur, loss of fracture reduction is a potential complication. Although it provides biomechanical stability, fragment-specific fixation cannot, in itself, always prevent collapse, and therefore diligent use of bone graft may be utilized [17]. Using fragment-specific fixation, Gavaskar et al. found a loss of reduction in 5/105 patients, four of whom had unaddressed dorsal comminution and one patient with volar carpal subluxation [31].

Conclusion

Fractures of the distal radius are common injuries, and with an expanding active elderly population with exceedingly high expectations to return to pre-injury activities, an increasing number of these fractures is being treated operatively. With recent advances in design, the great majority of these are treated with a volar plate. While one single approach to distal radius fractures is appealing due to its simplicity and ease of application, it has become clear that no single technique or implant can be the panacea to treat all variations of distal radius fractures. For comminuted intra-articular fractures, fragment-specific fixation can be utilized to achieve anatomic reduction. Fragment-specific fixation may seem daunting given the fixation options, but it provides an invaluable addition to a surgeon's armamentarium when faced with complex intra-articular fractures of the distal radius. Thus this technique, not a specific implant, must be kept in the toolbox of any surgeon taking care of patients with wrist fractures.

References

1. Cohen MS, Frillman T. Distal radius fractures: a prospective randomized comparison of fibreglass tape with QuickCast. Injury. 1997;28(4):305–9.
2. McKay SD, et al. Assessment of complications of distal radius fractures and development of a complication checklist. J Hand Surg Am. 2001;26(5):916–22.
3. Colles A. On the fracture of the carpal extremity of the radius. Edinb Med Surg J. 1814;10:181. Clin Orthop Relat Res. 2006;445:5–7.
4. Frykman G. Fracture of the distal radius including sequelae–shoulder-hand-finger syndrome, disturbance in the distal radio-ulnar joint and impairment of nerve function. A clinical and experimental study. Acta Orthop Scand. 1967;Suppl 108:3+.
5. Gartland Jr JJ, Werley CW. Evaluation of healed Colles' fractures. J Bone Joint Surg Am. 1951;33-A(4):895–907.
6. Chung KC, Spilson SV. The frequency and epidemiology of hand and forearm fractures in the United States. J Hand Surg Am. 2001;26(5): 908–15.
7. Kopylov P, et al. Fractures of the distal end of the radius in young adults: a 30-year follow-up. J Hand Surg Br. 1993;18(1):45–9.
8. Knirk JL, Jupiter JB. Intra-articular fractures of the distal end of the radius in young adults. J Bone Joint Surg Am. 1986;68(5):647–59.
9. Trumble TE, Schmitt SR, Vedder NB. Factors affecting functional outcome of displaced intra-articular distal radius fractures. J Hand Surg Am. 1994;19(2):325–40.
10. Ring D, et al. Prospective multicenter trial of a plate for dorsal fixation of distal radius fractures. J Hand Surg Am. 1997;22(5):777–84.
11. Ruch DS, Papadonikolakis A. Volar versus dorsal plating in the management of intra-articular distal radius fractures. J Hand Surg Am. 2006;31(1):9–16.
12. Simic PM, et al. Treatment of distal radius fractures with a low-profile dorsal plating system: an outcomes assessment. J Hand Surg Am. 2006;31(3):382–6.
13. Kamath AF, Zurakowski D, Day CS. Low-profile dorsal plating for dorsally angulated distal radius fractures: an outcomes study. J Hand Surg Am. 2006;31(7):1061–7.
14. Wright TW, Horodyski M, Smith DW. Functional outcome of unstable distal radius fractures: ORIF with a volar fixed-angle tine plate versus external fixation. J Hand Surg Am. 2005;30(2):289–99.
15. Freeland AE, Luber KT. Biomechanics and biology of plate fixation of distal radius fractures. Hand Clin. 2005;21(3):329–39.
16. Lucas GL, Fejfar ST. Complications in internal fixation of the distal radius. J Hand Surg Am. 1998;23(6):1117.
17. Schumer ED, Leslie BM. Fragment-specific fixation of distal radius fractures using the Trimed device. Tech Hand Up Extrem Surg. 2005; 9(2):74–83.

18. Konrath GA, Bahler S. Open reduction and internal fixation of unstable distal radius fractures: results using the trimed fixation system. J Orthop Trauma. 2002;16(8):578–85.
19. Benson LS, Medoff RJ. Fragment-specific fixation of distal radius fractures. In: Slutsky D.J, Osterman AL editors. Fractures and injuries of the distal radius and carpus. Philadelphia: W.B. Saunders; 2009.
20. Melone Jr CP. Articular fractures of the distal radius. Orthop Clin North Am. 1984;15(2):217–36.
21. Andersen DJ, et al. Classification of distal radius fractures: an analysis of interobserver reliability and intraobserver reproducibility. J Hand Surg Am. 1996;21(4):574–82.
22. Rikli DA, Regazzoni P. Fractures of the distal end of the radius treated by internal fixation and early function. A preliminary report of 20 cases. J Bone Joint Surg Br. 1996;78(4):588–92.
23. Leslie BMMRJ. Fracture specific fixation of distal radius fractures. Tech Orthop. 2000;15:336–52.
24. Bae DS, Koris MJ. Fragment-specific internal fixation of distal radius fractures. Hand Clin. 2005;21(3):355–62.
25. Dodds SD, et al. A biomechanical comparison of fragment-specific fixation and augmented external fixation for intra-articular distal radius fractures. J Hand Surg Am. 2002;27(6):953–64.
26. Harness NG, et al. Loss of fixation of the volar lunate facet fragment in fractures of the distal part of the radius. J Bone Joint Surg Am. 2004;86-A(9):1900–8.
27. Swigart CR, Wolfe SW. Limited incision open techniques for distal radius fracture management. Orthop Clin North Am. 2001;32(2):317–27. ix.
28. Taylor KF, Parks BG, Segalman KA. Biomechanical stability of a fixed-angle volar plate versus fragment-specific fixation system: cyclic testing in a C2-type distal radius cadaver fracture model. J Hand Surg Am. 2006;31(3):373–81.
29. Cooper EO, et al. Biomechanical stability of a volar locking-screw plate versus fragment-specific fixation in a distal radius fracture model. Am J Orthop (Belle Mead NJ). 2007;36(4):E46–9.
30. Benson LS, et al. The outcome of intra-articular distal radius fractures treated with fragment-specific fixation. J Hand Surg Am. 2006;31(8):1333–9.
31. Gavaskar AS, Muthukumar S, Chowdary N. Fragment-specific fixation for complex intra-articular fractures of the distal radius: results of a prospective single-centre trial. J Hand Surg Eur Vol. 2012;37(8):765–71.
32. Meyer C, et al. Complications of distal radial and scaphoid fracture treatment. Instr Course Lect. 2014;63:113–22.

Chapter 8
Volar Ulnar Fixation

Varun K. Gajendran and Kevin J. Malone

Case Presentation

A healthy, active 43-year-old right-hand dominant female presented 2 days after a fall with right wrist pain, swelling, and mild deformity. She had been initially treated at an outside facility with a short arm splint. She had no neurologic symptoms and her neurovascular examination was within normal limits. Radiographs (Fig. 8.1a, b) demonstrated a distal radius fracture with a minimally displaced radial styloid fragment and a significantly displaced volar lunate facet fragment. Axial (Fig. 8.1c) and sagittal (Fig. 8.1d) cuts of a computed tomography (CT) scan revealed the volar lunate facet fragment to be significantly displaced volarly and ulnarly.

Given the large amount of displacement of the volar lunate facet, we recommended surgical reduction and fixation of the fracture. Based upon the location, the fracture was approached through an extended carpal tunnel incision just ulnar to the palmaris longus and the transverse carpal ligament was released (Fig. 8.1e).

V.K. Gajendran, MD (✉) • K.J. Malone, MD
Department of Orthopaedic Surgery, MetroHealth Medical Center,
2500 MetroHealth Drive, Cleveland, OH 44109, USA
e-mail: varun182@gmail.com

© Springer International Publishing Switzerland 2016   89
J.N. Lawton (ed.), *Distal Radius Fractures*,
DOI 10.1007/978-3-319-27489-8_8

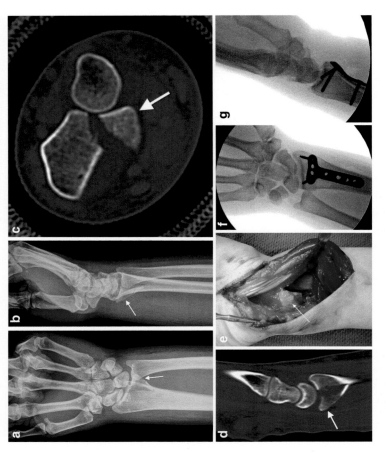

Fig. 8.1 A 43-year-old female fell and sustained a distal radius fracture with a minimally displaced but comminuted radial styloid and a volarly and ulnarly displaced volar lunate facet (*white arrow*), as shown on the AP (**a**) and lateral (**b**) injury films, as well as CT axial (**c**) and sagittal (**d**) cuts; the fracture was approached through an extended carpal tunnel incision (**e**), and anatomically reduced and fixed with a 2.7 mm buttress T-plate (**f**, **g**)

The superficial and deep flexor tendons were then retracted radially with the median nerve, while the flexor carpi ulnaris and ulnar neurovascular bundle were retracted ulnarly, providing excellent access to the displaced volar lunate facet fragment (Fig. 8.1e). The fracture was anatomically reduced and fixed with a 2.7 mm T-plate in buttress mode (Fig. 8.1f, g).

That patient was immobilized in a short arm splint for 2 weeks, followed by a short arm cast for 4 weeks, and serial X-rays were obtained during her regularly scheduled clinic visits. Her postoperative course was uncomplicated. At her final follow-up of 6 months post-operatively, she had no pain and had returned to all activities. She had full range of motion of her wrist and forearm with excellent grip strength, and radiographs showed a healed fracture and a reduced DRUJ.

Discussion

With any distal radius fracture, it is critical to evaluate the status of the volar lunate facet for three important reasons. Firstly, it constitutes the intermediate column of the wrist and is the most important load-bearing portion of the distal radial articular surface, and therefore a near-anatomic reduction is desirable [1]. Secondly, it articulates with the sigmoid notch to form the volar aspect of the distal radioulnar joint (DRUJ), which is important for normal wrist and forearm rotation. Lastly, and perhaps most importantly, it is normally attached to the short radiocarpal ligament, an important volar extrinsic ligament that plays a vital role in maintaining radiocarpal stability [2–6].

Although volar locking plates have generally been very effective in dealing with traditionally difficult fracture patterns with low complication rates, failure of fixation can still be a problem [7, 8]. In particular, many studies have demonstrated the challenges of obtaining reduction and fixation of the critical volar lunate facet even in experienced hands due to the often small size and comminuted nature of the fragment [5, 6, 9]. Beck et al. noted that even perfectly positioned volar locking plates risked loss of fixation and radiocarpal subsidence when the lunate facet fragment was less than 15 mm in size or there was greater than 5 mm of initial lunate subsidence [10]. Critical evaluation preoperatively must take this volar ulnar fragment size into account to ensure that the selected plate will appropriately provide fixation.

Malreduction of the volar lunate facet fragment can lead to limitation of forearm rotation and DRUJ arthrosis. Loss of fixation of the fragment can lead to the disastrous complication of radio-carpal dislocation, which can be extremely challenging to treat if not recognized immediately [5, 6, 9, 10]. To address these potential problems, numerous techniques have been developed, ranging from percutaneous to arthroscopic-assisted to open, and utilizing a variety of implants including headless screws, external fixation combined with internal fixation, volar locking plates designed specifically to buttress and capture the volar lunate facet fragment, and fragment-specific fixation with mini-plates, hook plates, figure-8 tension-band, and wire-form fixation [2, 3, 6, 11–21].

Our Approach

In addition to the normal workup for a distal radius fracture, there are specific characteristics of this injury that require special attention on history and physical examination. Displaced volar ulnar fragments are often the result of high-energy trauma, and the patient should be questioned about median nerve symptoms. Contusions are common due to the location of the median nerve directly overlying the volar lunate facet, and acute carpal tunnel syndrome can also occur from fracture hematoma or direct compression of the median nerve by a displaced lunate facet fragment [22]. While contusions occur from the moment of impact during injury and remain symptomatically stable, acute carpal tunnel syndrome is distinguished by the progression of symptoms over time and should be treated urgently with surgical release. Fracture fixation is generally performed simultaneously to provide early stabilization.

Plain radiographs should be studied closely to ensure that the teardrop, which represents the volar lunate facet and can be seen projecting anteriorly on the lateral X-ray, is normal in appearance and orientation. Incorrect orientation alone, even without much displacement, can be a clue to the fragment being significantly rotated on the short radiolunate ligament pedicle distally, and this warrants reduction and fixation of the fragment to restore radiocarpal and radioulnar stability [23, 24]. The posteroanterior (PA) radiograph should also be examined to ensure the normal orientation of the dorsal articular margin of the lunate facet being slightly more distal than the volar articular margin due to the normal volar tilt of the articular surface [24, 25]. The volar lunate facet fragment is created by the transmission of energy between the long and short radiolunate ligaments at their insertions on the distal radius, and the scapholunate interval, which is also in this path, should also be assessed for injury. A post-reduction X-ray or traction X-ray will often better demonstrate the volar lunate facet, which may be obscured on the injury films by bone overlap. Although we do not routinely perform advanced imaging, a computed tomography (CT) of the wrist is often useful in this fracture pattern to study the size and orientation of the individual fragments including the volar lunate facet, and it can also aid with pre-operative planning.

Whenever we encounter a distal radius fracture with a significantly displaced volar lunate facet, or one that is small or comminuted and poses a real risk of loss of fixation with volar locked plating alone, we consider addressing it with a separate implant. Accurate reduction and secure fixation of this fragment is critical to restoring radiocarpal and radioulnar stability [5, 6, 9, 10, 15, 26]. We evaluate the status of this fragment in conjunction with the other fractured fragments and develop a plan that involves volar locked plating alone with screws through the plate into the volar lunate facet fragment or fragment-specific fixation with a separate implant for the volar lunate facet combined with a radial styloid plate, dorsal plate, spanning plate, and/or external fixation.

If we need to directly access and manipulate the volar lunate facet fragment, we often utilize an extended carpal tunnel incision just ulnar to the palmaris longus and concurrently perform a carpal tunnel release distally as part of the procedure given the high associated risk of developing acute carpal tunnel syndrome [22]. In these cases, we combine our extended carpal tunnel incision

with a radial-sided incision to fix the radial styloid fragment and/
or a dorsal incision to address any dorsal fragments when necessary. If, on the other hand, the volar ulnar fragment is large and
minimally displaced, we perform a more typical Henry volar
approach through the interval between the flexor carpi radialis and
radial artery, and broadly elevate the pronator quadratus on its
ulnar pedicle to allow us to access the volar lunate facet for reduction and fixation with screws through a volar locking plate. Care
must be taken, however, as the contents of the carpal must be
retracted with broad retractors.

When utilizing fragment-specific fixation, the volar lunate
facet can be fixed with wire-form fixation or small T- or L-shaped
2.0, 2.4, or 2.7 mm locking plates functioning in buttress mode.
K-wires and mini-fragment screws can be used to augment the
fixation, but should not be used alone. For fragments that are too
small to support plate/screw constructs, the volar capsule and
short radiolunate ligament can be captured with a #2 Ethibond
horizontal mattress or modified Kessler stitch and this can be
repaired to the intact distal radius just proximal to the fracture
through drill holes in the volar cortex. This technique can also be
used with plate fixation for added reinforcement. Locking plates
are preferred, with non-locking screws inserted first proximal to
the fracture to buttress the volar lunate facet fragment, followed
by locking screws into the fragment itself after elevation and bone
grafting of the articular surface as necessary to prevent displacement, rotation, and subsidence.

Tips and Tricks

The key to successful reduction and fixation of the volar ulnar corner is adequate pre-operative planning that anticipates the characteristics of the fracture and accordingly selects the appropriate
exposure and implants as described above. A small, rolled towel
bump placed dorsally under the distal forearm can help translate
the proximal fragment volarly to aid in the reduction. After

exposure, the fragment should be gently manipulated with pick-ups, dental picks, and small K-wires acting as joysticks. Bone clamps can be used for larger fragments, but they can crush and destabilize smaller fragments, particularly when the bone is osteopenic. Figure 8.2 illustrates one such case of a small volar ulnar fragment that poses unique challenges for reduction and fixation. The fragment's soft tissue attachments consisting of the capsule and volar extrinsic ligaments should be preserved to maintain its vascularity and also radiocarpal stability after fixation. If the reduction seems difficult, the surgeon must keep in mind that these fragments can often be rotated 180° around the distal insertion of the short radiolunate ligament on the lunate.

The reduced volar ulnar fragment can usually be held in place with a dental pick while a 0.045-inch K-wire is inserted into it for provisional fixation, starting at the volar distal apex of the teardrop and going proximally into the dorsal cortex of the metaphysis. The K-wire should be placed in a location that does not interfere with eventual plate placement. The distal aspect of the plate should extend to the distal extent of the volar lip to block and prevent volar escape of small volar ulnar fragments. The distal aspect of the plate should be pre-bent to exactly match the contour of the volar lip, but the part of the plate that is just proximal to the fracture can be purposely under-contoured to allow the screw just proximal to the fracture to push the plate against the volar cortex to achieve a greater buttress effect. This screw should be inserted first, followed by one more screw proximally. Screws do not need to be inserted into the distal fragment through the plate if the distal aspect of the plate adequately stabilizes the fracture through a buttress effect. If possible, however, locking screws should be inserted through the distal plates holes to provide added stability to the construct. They will generally need to be aimed slightly proximally to avoid articular penetration, and this may be done under fluoroscopy. One must keep in mind that plates in this area are by definition distal to the watershed line and may therefore irritate the flexor tendons, so any measures to reduce the bulkiness of the implant distal to the watershed area should be considered [27]. In addition to the plate, K-wires, mini-fragment screws, headless

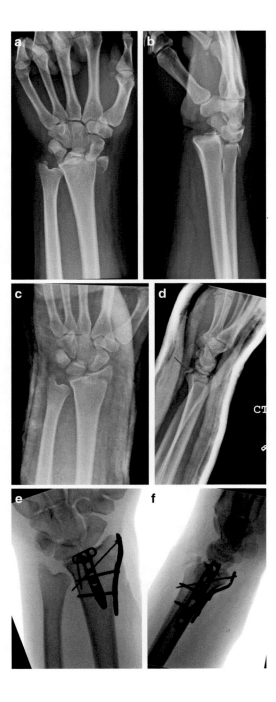

screws, or suture through the capsule and volar extrinsic ligaments can be used to augment the fixation. Any fixation distal to the watershed line will be an irritant to the flexor tendons, a planned hardware removal as a second stage must be discussed with the patient.

After fixation has been performed, a gentle stress radiograph should be obtained by attempting to translate the hand with the volar lunate facet fragment volarly to ensure that the radiocarpal joint remains well-reduced. The stability of the DRUJ, as well as rotation, should be assessed to ensure that there is no malreduction of the volar ulnar fragment or other DRUJ injury. Lastly, the scapholunate interval should be checked with an ulnar deviated PA view to assess for dynamic instability. Although the treatment of these additional injuries is beyond the scope of this chapter, they should be treated appropriately after fracture fixation.

Post-operatively, the patient should be placed in a forearm based splint that leaves the metacarpophalangeal (MP) joints free. The patient should be followed-up in clinic weekly for the first 2–3 weeks with X-rays to ensure no loss of fixation or reduction. At the 2-week post-operative visit, sutures can be removed and the patient can be placed in a short arm cast. The cast should be worn for an additional 4 weeks, and pending appropriate healing, gentle wrist motion is begun at this time, with strengthening initiated at around 12 weeks.

Fig. 8.2 Injury AP (**a**) and lateral (**b**) views of the wrist of a 21-year-old male involved in a motorcycle accident show a high-energy distal radius fracture with dorsal radiocarpal dislocation and a small associated radial styloid fracture, and post-reduction AP (**c**) and lateral (**d**) X-rays reveal interval reduction with a teardrop representing the volar lunate facet (*white arrow*) that is rotated 180° from its normal orientation; this was approached through an extended carpal tunnel incision and the volar lunate facet was fixed with a 2.4 mm buttress T-plate and a 0.045-inch K-wire, and the radial styloid was approached through a separate radial incision and fixed with a 2.4 mm radial styloid plate and a 0.045-inch K-wire (**e, f**)

References

1. Rikli DA, Regazzoni P. Fractures of the distal end of the radius treated by internal fixation and early function. A preliminary report of 20 cases. J Bone Joint Surg Br. 1996;78(4):588–92.
2. Bakker AJ, Shin AY. Fragment-specific volar hook plate for volar marginal rim fractures. Tech Hand Up Extrem Surg. 2014;18(1):56–60.
3. Bae DS, Koris MJ. Fragment-specific internal fixation of distal radius fractures. Hand Clin. 2005;21(3):355–62.
4. Berger RA, Landsmeer JM. The palmar radiocarpal ligaments: a study of adult and fetal human wrist joints. J Hand Surg Am. 1990;15(6):847–54.
5. Kitay A, Mudgal C. Volar carpal subluxation following lunate facet fracture. J Hand Surg Am. 2014;39(11):2335–41.
6. Harness NG, Jupiter JB, Orbay JL, et al. Loss of fixation of the volar lunate facet fragment in fractures of the distal part of the radius. J Bone Joint Surg Am. 2004;86-A(9):1900–8.
7. Soong M, van Leerdam R, Guitton TG, et al. Fracture of the distal radius: risk factors for complications after locked volar plate fixation. J Hand Surg Am. 2011;36(1):3–9.
8. Rozental TD, Blazar PE. Functional outcome and complications after volar plating for dorsally displaced, unstable fractures of the distal radius. J Hand Surg Am. 2006;31(3):359–65.
9. Tan KG, Chew WY. Beware! The volar ulnar fragment in a comminuted Bartons fracture. Hand Surg. 2013;18(3):331–6.
10. Beck JD, Harness NG, Spencer HT. Volar plate fixation failure for volar shearing distal radius fractures with small lunate facet fragments. J Hand Surg Am. 2014;39(4):670–8.
11. Benson LS, Minihane KP, Stern LD, et al. The outcome of intra-articular distal radius fractures treated with fragment-specific fixation. J Hand Surg Am. 2006;31(8):1333–9.
12. Chin KR, Jupiter JB. Wire-loop fixation of volar displaced osteochondral fractures of the distal radius. J Hand Surg Am. 1999;24(3):525–33.
13. Dodds SD, Cornelissen S, Jossan S, et al. A biomechanical comparison of fragment-specific fixation and augmented external fixation for intra-articular distal radius fractures. J Hand Surg Am. 2002;27(6):953–64.
14. Geissler WB, Fernandes D. Percutaneous and limited open reduction of intra-articular distal radial fractures. Hand Surg. 2000;5(2):85–92.
15. Martineau PA, Waitayawinyu T, Malone KJ, et al. Volar plating of AO C3 distal radius fractures: biomechanical evaluation of locking screw and locking smooth peg configurations. J Hand Surg Am. 2008;33(6):827–34.
16. Moore AM, Dennison DG. Distal radius fractures and the volar lunate facet fragment: Kirschner wire fixation in addition to volar-locked plating. Hand (N Y). 2014;9(2):230–6.
17. Ring D, Jupiter JB. Percutaneous and limited open fixation of fractures of the distal radius. Clin Orthop Relat Res. 2000;(375):105–15.

18. Ruch DS, Yang C, Smith BP. Results of palmar plating of the lunate facet combined with external fixation for the treatment of high-energy compression fractures of the distal radius. J Orthop Trauma. 2004;18(1):28–33.

19. Saw N, Roberts C, Cutbush K, et al. Early experience with the TriMed fragment-specific fracture fixation system in intraarticular distal radius fractures. J Hand Surg Eur Vol. 2008;33(1):53–8.

20. Waters MJ, Ruchelsman DE, Belsky MR, et al. Headless bone screw fixation for combined volar lunate facet distal radius fracture and capitate fracture: case report. J Hand Surg Am. 2014;39(8):1489–93.

21. Wiesler ER, Chloros GD, Lucas RM, et al. Arthroscopic management of volar lunate facet fractures of the distal radius. Tech Hand Up Extrem Surg. 2006;10(3):139–44.

22. Paley D, McMurtry RY. Median nerve compression by volarly displaced fragments of the distal radius. Clin Orthop Relat Res. 1987;(215):139–47.

23. Fujitani R, Omokawa S, Iida A, et al. Reliability and clinical importance of teardrop angle measurement in intra-articular distal radius fracture. J Hand Surg Am. 2012;37(3):454–9.

24. Medoff RJ. Essential radiographic evaluation for distal radius fractures. Hand Clin. 2005;21(3):279–88.

25. Andermahr J, Lozano-Calderon S, Trafton T, et al. The volar extension of the lunate facet of the distal radius: a quantitative anatomic study. J Hand Surg Am. 2006;31(6):892–5.

26. Rampoldi M, Marsico S. Complications of volar plating of distal radius fractures. Acta Orthop Belg. 2007;73(6):714–9.

27. Soong M, Earp BE, Bishop G, et al. Volar locking plate implant prominence and flexor tendon rupture. J Bone Joint Surg Am. 2011;93(4):328–35.

Chapter 9
Fractures of the Radial Column

Eitan Melamed and Dawn M. LaPorte

Case Presentation

A 66-year-old right hand dominant female fell from a standing height onto her outstretched hand. She sustained a displaced left radial styloid fracture. There was no evidence of carpal subluxation or scapholunate malalignment on initial X-rays (Fig. 9.1). The lunate facet appeared to remain reduced relative to the proximal radius, and it was therefore decided to reconstruct the injury back to the stable reference point of the lunate facet. During the initial reduction, however, it was noted that the lunate facet fragment was unstable, requiring rigid fixation (Fig. 9.2), making it a three-part fracture. Treatment included open reduction and internal fixation of the radial column through a dorsal radial approach, using a 2.4 mm dorsal distal radius plate (Synthes, Paoli, USA), followed

E. Melamed, MD
Department of Plastic Surgery, Johns Hopkins Medical Center,
Johns Hopkins Bayview Medical Center, 4940 Eastern Ave.,
Room A 518, Baltimore, MD 21224, USA
e-mail: eitanme2000@yahoo.com

D.M. LaPorte, MD (✉)
Orthopaedic Surgery, Johns Hopkins University School of Medicine,
601 North Caroline Street, Baltimore, MD 21287, USA
e-mail: dlaport1@jhmi.edu

© Springer International Publishing Switzerland 2016   101
J.N. Lawton (ed.), *Distal Radius Fractures*,
DOI 10.1007/978-3-319-27489-8_9

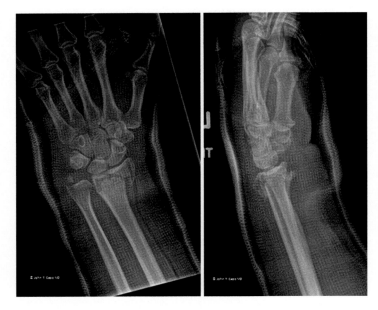

Fig. 9.1 Preoperative X-rays (*Courtesy of Dr John Capo*)

by an ulnar column plate through a separate approach (Fig. 9.3a). At 5 weeks (Fig. 9.3b), the patient had no pain over the radial styloid and had full and symmetric range-of-motion compared to the contralateral extremity.

Introduction

Fractures of the radial column may be relatively simple, isolated distal radius fractures, a component of a more complex distal radius fracture or part of an incomplete or complete greater arc perilunate dislocation, involving intrinsic and extrinsic carpal ligaments (Fig. 9.4). This is highlighted by the fact that scapholunate (SL) ligament injuries were noted in 50 % of displaced distal radius fractures in non-osteoporotic patients [1], making this injury more than a "distal radius fracture." When evaluating radial

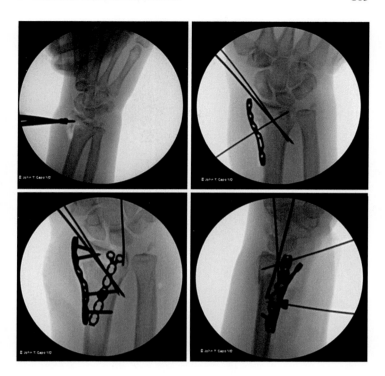

Fig. 9.2 Intraoperative X-rays showing initial reduction maneuver and provisional fixation of the radial column fragment. During reduction, a displaced volar lunate facet fragment was noticed. Lunate facet plating was performed in order to stabilize the volar fragment (*Courtesy of Dr John Capo*)

column fractures, one must therefore rule out concomitant ligament injuries, because the sequelae of failing to treat associated injuries can result in long-term wrist degeneration [2].

Anatomy

The radial column is a bony buttress that supports the scaphoid fossa and serves as attachment for the extrinsic carpal ligaments [3]. The radial styloid is the palpable bony prominence on the radial side of the wrist. The superficial branch of the radial nerve (SBRN)

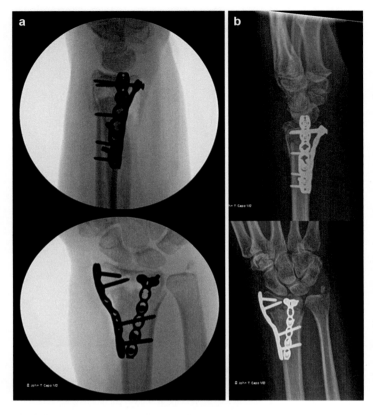

Fig. 9.3 Immediate (**a**) and 5 weeks (**b**) postoperative X-rays. Note the relatively volar position of the radial column plate, with the plates not appearing parallel (*Courtesy of Dr John Capo*)

lies in the subcutaneous fat immediately under the skin, just proximal to the radial styloid (Fig. 9.5). The palmar branch of the SBRN divides before the main nerve passes over the first dorsal compartment. A safe zone for K-wire insertion at the radial styloid has been defined, bordered proximally by the styloid tip, distally by the radial artery, dorsally by the dorsal trunk of SBRN, and volarly by the first dorsal compartment [4]. Therefore, a 1 cm incision is recommended distal to the tip of the radial styloid before K-wire insertion. The tendons of the first dorsal compartment are located within

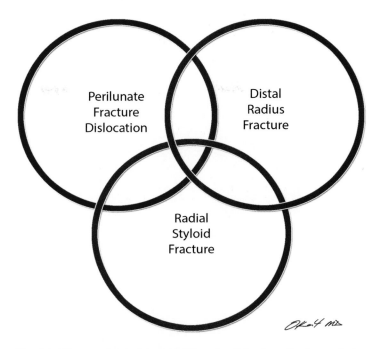

Fig. 9.4 Diagram showing the variability of radial column fractures, placing them in context as either isolated, part of a more complex fracture pattern or as a component of perilunate fracture dislocation (carpal instability or radiocarpal dislocation)

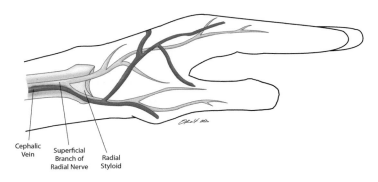

Fig. 9.5 Illustration showing the course of the SBRN and cephalic vein relative to the radial styloid

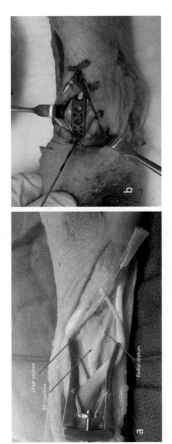

Fig. 9.6 Cadaver dissection showing (**a**) radial septum for abductor pollicis brevis, brachioradialis (BR) tendon insertion, and radial styloid (needle); and (**b**) radial column plate placed in the floor of the first dorsal compartment between the septums. The BR needs to be dissected off the radial styloid to facilitate reduction and allow access for fixation

two fibro-osseous septums, on the volar radial and dorsal radial aspects of the radial styloid (Fig. 9.6a) with the brachioradialis lying on the floor of the compartment. The space between the septums can accommodate radial column plates (Fig. 9.6b).

Radiology

Routine radiographic views should include posteroanterior (PA), true lateral and 45° pronated view. On the PA view, the radial styloid is visualized in profile and, on the lateral view, the styloid has a curved appearance superimposed on the lunate. Critical review of the lateral may demonstrate translation—often missed upon casual glance. The 45° pronated view best demonstrates radial styloid fractures which are not always appreciated in the standard frontal PA and lateral views where the styloid may appear relatively normal [5]. Since radial styloid fracture may represent a part of a greater arc perilunate injury, its presence should lead the surgeon to suspect a high grade SL ligament injury. The best view to evaluate the SL joint is the supinated AP view [6]. Clenched fist views are useful for demonstrating instability but may be impossible to obtain with acute fractures. Instead, stress views are obtained in the operating room following fixation of the bony elements. The wrist is moved into radial and ulnar deviation and widening of the SL joint is noted. MRI scans are useful in detecting ligament injuries, but have a poor interobserver reliability [7]. A negative MRI on its own is insufficient to exclude a structural ligament injury. The combination of physical examination, radiographs, and arthroscopy is an excellent method of evaluating ligament integrity [8].

Mechanism of Injury

Radial column fractures have been termed in the past "chauffer's fractures" [9] due to the early description of the fracture resulting from backfire of the automobile's crank in the early twentieth century. Today, the majority of radial-sided wrist injuries occur from a fall on an outstretched hand. The resultant axial and hyperextension load will lead to either distal radius or scaphoid fracture. If the mechanism of injury combines hyperextension, ulnar deviation, and intercarpal supination, progressive perilunate fracture dislocation will occur [10]. The injury begins at the radial aspect of the wrist and propagates towards the ulnar side through the midcarpal space. The lesser arc injury involves the intercarpal and intrinsic ligaments without an associated fracture. The greater arc injury involves a fracture of one or more carpal bones and disruption of the midcarpal articulation, of which the most common type is trans-scaphoid dorsal perilunate fracture dislocation. An inferior arc injury is propagated through the radiocarpal joint instead of traversing the carpus. The extrinsic ligaments on the volar and dorsal aspects may be disrupted and/or a fracture of the radial styloid may occur. When the force propagates through the tip of the radial styloid, it may cause avulsion of the radioscaphocapitate (RSC) ligament, allowing ulnar carpal translation. The force then propagates through the extrinsic radiocarpal ligaments, resulting in radiocarpal dislocation. *The combination of radial and ulnar styloid fractures should raise suspicion for this potentially unstable injury.*

If, however, the force propagates from a more proximal location on the radial column through the scapholunate ridge of the distal radius, there is a high risk of SL ligament injury (Fig. 9.7), as well as other components of perilunate injury.

Classification

The AO classification divides distal radius fractures into extraarticular type A, partial-articular type B, and complete-articular type C fractures [11]. Radial column fractures fall under type B as follows:

B1.1: simple radial styloid fracture
B1.2: multifragmentary radial styloid fracture

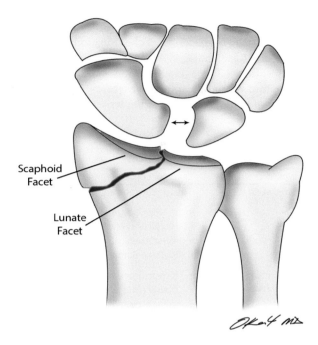

Fig. 9.7 Radial column fracture with an associated SL ligament injury, highlighting that the spectrum of perilunate injuries can involve radial-sided structures only without full blown perilunate dislocation

B 2.2: more complex radiocarpal fracture subluxation that includes a radial styloid fragment

B 2.3: high-energy radiocarpal dorsal fracture dislocation with a radial styloid fracture, comminuted dorsal rim, and disruption of the DRUJ.

Perilunate fracture dislocations have been further classified [12], where styloid tip fractures are referred to as associated chip fractures and fractures through the base of the radial styloid represent a subgroup of greater arc perilunate fracture dislocation. Dumontier et al. [13] classified radiocarpal dislocations into 2 groups. Group 1 is defined as either pure dislocation or a dislocation with an associated radial styloid tip avulsion. Group 2 is a radiocarpal dislocation with an associated fracture of the radial styloid involving greater than one-third of the scaphoid fossa. Green and O'Brien [14] described a classification for carpal dislocations and included radial styloid fractures as a subgroup of carpal dislocations. These classification systems highlight the complex nature of radial column fractures, placing them on the spectrum of complex injuries to the wrist.

Table 9.1 Working classification for radial column fractures and treatment options

Fracture type	Treatment options
Isolated radial styloid fracture	Closed reduction and casting • K-wire fixation • Headless screw fixation • Volar plate • Radial column plate
Radial styloid fractures as part of a distal radius fracture	• K-wire fixation • Dorsal plate • Volar plate • Combined volar and radial fixation with either radial column plate/K-wires/headless screw • External fixation
Radial styloid and scaphoid fractures	• Casting (if completely nondisplaced) • K-wire fixation • Headless screw fixation • Volar plate • Radial column plate
Radial styloid fractures with carpal instability	• Open reduction of carpal malalignment • Anatomic reduction and fixation of the radial styloid
Radial styloid fractures with radiocarpal dislocation	• Radiocarpal reduction • Open anatomic reduction and fixation of the radial styloid • Possible volar radiocarpal ligament repair for radial styloid tip avulsion fractures
Radial styloid fractures with translunate fractures	• Lunate fracture stabilization • Radial styloid stabilization with K-wires/headless screws

A simple working classification presented by Reichel et al. [2] and based on the concomitant injuries puts the fracture in the proper context and guides the treatment (Table 9.1).

Treatment

Nonsurgical Treatment

The truly nondisplaced radial styloid fracture can be treated nonoperatively, after thorough radiographic evaluation including 45° pronated PA view. This fracture should be carefully followed by weekly radiographs due to its inherently unstable nature. Even a nondisplaced radial styloid fracture can displace later as a result of the pull of the brachioradialis on the styloid fragment. If one chooses closed treatment, immobilization in supination should be considered, due to the lower muscle activity of the brachioradialis in this position [15].

Surgical Treatment

Radial Styloid Tip Fracture

Styloid tip fractures are typically extraarticular and should always be evaluated for associated radiocarpal instability (Dumontier group 1). The extrinsic radiocarpal ligaments are tested under fluoroscopy, as the hand and carpus are shifted versus the forearm, both ulnarly and in the sagittal plane. If more than 6–8 mm of the styloid tip is involved, the RSC ligament is avulsed with the bone but still connected to the fragment. That may portend a better prognosis than tip fractures, as anatomic reduction and fixation will usually result in bony union and establish radiocarpal stability.

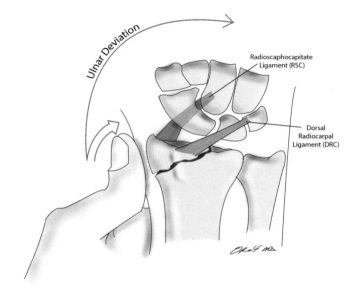

Fig. 9.8 Closed reduction of radial styloid fractures

Simple Radial Styloid Base Fractures

These fractures are typically intra-articular and should be considered for surgery if articular incongruity is greater than 2 mm [16]. Treatment alternatives include closed reduction and casting, K-wire fixation, headless screw fixation, volar plate, and radial column plate. Displaced radial styloid base fractures are inherently unstable, and as such they are best treated with stable internal fixation. Closed reduction and K-wire fixation are often sufficient. The reduction maneuver involves direct thumb pressure over the styloid with ulnar deviation (Fig. 9.8). Alternatively, K-wires can be percutaneously introduced into the styloid and used as joysticks to reduce the fracture and overcome the pull of the brachioradialis. An oscillating drill is used to insert K-wires into the radial styloid, or if a small skin incision is made, a protective sleeve is used to avoid damage to the SBRN (Fig. 9.9).

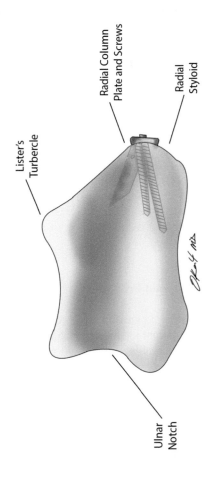

Fig. 9.9 Trapezoidal profile of the distal radius, showing the relatively palmar location of the radial styloid, and screw trajectory in 50°–90° of offset in the axial plane, relative to the dorsal-ulnar plane

If the fracture cannot be reduced closed, an open approach is required. The open approach to the radial column is either a dorso-radial approach or a volar approach. The dorsoradial is performed through a longitudinal dorsoradial incision between the first and second dorsal compartments, with release of the proximal portion of the first dorsal compartment retinaculum. The brachioradialis is dissected off the bone to allow reduction and hardware placement. The SBRN is protected at all times. The volar radial approach uses the interval between the radial artery and the first dorsal compartment [17]. Definitive fixation methods include K-wires, headless screws, and fragment-specific radial column plates. There are no comparative outcome studies for isolated radial column fractures favoring one fixation method over another. If screws are used, they should be inserted perpendicular to the fracture plane to maximize compression (Fig. 9.10). If a radial column plate is used, it is placed between the first and second dorsal compartments, with the screws in 50°–90° of offset in the axial plane, to the dorsal-ulnar plane (Fig. 9.9). An effort should be made to prevent hardware prominence over cortical bone and reduce the risk of tendon and nerve irritation.

Comminuted Radial Styloid Fractures

These fractures are usually a part of a more complex distal radius fracture. Acceptable treatment modalities include K-wire fixation, dorsal plate, volar plate, combined volar and radial fixation with either radial column plate, K-wires or a headless screw and external fixation. The surgical approach depends on fracture geometry and whether additional volar or dorsal fixation is needed. Operative approaches include the dorsoradial approach between the first and second dorsal compartment and the standard volar FCR approach. A volar plate through the standard FCR approach can frequently allow secure fixation of a sizable styloid fragment, especially the more transversely oriented fractures (Fig. 9.11).

If the volar flexor carpi radialis approach is used for volar implant positioning, the dorsoradial approach can be performed concomitantly without the risk of vascular compromise to the intervening skin bridge because the radial artery lies within the

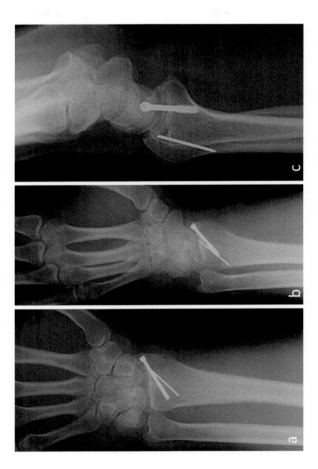

Fig. 9.10 Postoperative posteroanterior, oblique, and lateral radiographs of a displaced radial styloid fracture treated with an open reduction and headless internal fixation augmented with a K-wire (*Courtesy of Dr Scott Lifchez*)

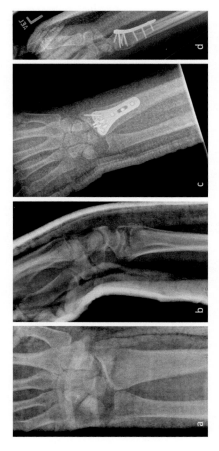

Fig. 9.11 Preoperative (**a**, **b**) and postoperative (**c**, **d**) posteroanterior and lateral views of a two-part radial styloid fracture treated with a volar plate. Note that the fracture line ends near the ridge between the radial and lunate fossae (**a**), and note the "ring sign" of the scaphoid, indicative of SL ligament injury (**c**) (*Courtesy of Dr Scott Lifchez*)

interval [18]. In a three-part articular fracture treated with a volar plate, additional screw fixation of the radial column significantly increased the stability of the construct and load to failure in a cadaver model [19].

In a randomized prospective trial comparing external fixation, radial column fixation, and volar plating for the treatment of unstable distal radius fractures with a 12-month follow-up, it was found that radial plating maintained radial inclination and radial height significantly better than external fixation and volar plate fixation. At 1 year, all patients had excellent reported outcomes [20]. In the absence of outcome studies comparing specific treatments for the radial styloid component, this study is important because it reports excellent functional results with a variety of treatment options for unstable distal radius fractures.

Complications

Percutaneous pinning has a reported complication rate of SBRN injuries of up to 20 % [21]. Using blunt dissection and drill sleeves can lower the risk of nerve injuries. Although the radial or dorsal radial approach may seem the most direct to the styloid, the small branches of the SBRN, which may be more susceptible to painful neuroma formation, are directly encountered with this approach. The more proximally the K-wires are inserted, the more likely they are to injure the main SBRN. Surgeons must be conscious of this when inserting the K-wire into a proximally displaced styloid component and when using K-wires to manipulate the component back into position. The safe zone for K-wire insertion has been defined on intact specimens where the styloid is in an anatomic unbroken position; this is not the case when K-wires are inserted before reduction. Placement of radial plates is possible from the volar approach and more likely to avoid injury to the SBRN, because the dissection is deep to the nerve and its branches.

References

1. Lindau T, Arner M, Hagberg L. Intraarticular lesions in distal fractures of the radius in young adults. A descriptive arthroscopic study in 50 patients. JHS. 1997;22B:63.
2. Reichel LM, Bell BR, Michnick SM, Reitman CA. Radial styloid fractures. J Hand Surg Am. 2012;37(8):1726–41.
3. Rikli DA, Regazzoni P. Fractures of the distal end of the radius treated by internal fixation and early function. A preliminary report of 20 cases. J Bone Joint Surg Br. 1996;78(4):588–92.
4. Steinberg BD, Plancher KD, Idler RS. Percutaneous Kirschner wire fixation through the snuff box: an anatomic study. J Hand Surg. 1995;20A:57–62.
5. Cohen M, Wysocki R. Fractures of the distal radius. In: Browner BD, Jupiter JB, Krettek, C, Anderson PA, editors. Skeletal trauma: basic science, management and reconstruction, Chapter 44. Philadelphia, PA: Saunders; 2015. p. 1263–1311.e5.
6. Taleisnik J. Current concepts review. Carpal instability. J Bone Joint Surg Am. 1988 Sep;70(8):1262–8.
7. Kuo CE, Wolfe SW. Scapholunate instability: current concepts in diagnosis and management. J Hand Surg Am. 2008;33(6):998–1013.
8. Henry M. Perilunate dislocations and fracture dislocations/radiocarpal dislocations and fracture dislocations. In: del Piñal F, Luchetti R, Mathoulin C, editors. Arthroscopic management of distal radius fractures, Chapter 11. Berlin: Springer; 2010. p. 127–49.
9. Stephens P. So-called chauffeur's fracture. Cal State J Med. 1923;21:115–7.
10. Mayfield JK, Johnson RP, Kilcoyne RK. Carpal dislocations: pathomechanics and progressive perilunar instability. J Hand Surg Am. 1980;5:226–41.
11. Müller ME, Nazarian S, Koch P, Schatzker J. AO classification of fractures. Berlin: Springer; 1987. p. 106–15.
12. Herzberg G, Comtet JJ, Linscheid RL, Amadio PC, Cooney WP, Stalder J. Perilunate dislocations and fracture-dislocations: a multicenter study. J Hand Surg Am. 1993;18:768–79.
13. Dumontier C, Meyerzu Reckendorf G, Sautet A, Lenoble E, Saffar P, Allieu Y. Radiocarpal dislocations: classification and proposal for treatment a review of twenty-seven cases. J Bone Joint Surg 2001;83A:212–8.
14. Green DP, O'Brien ET. Classification and management of carpal dislocations. Clin Orthop Relat Res. 1980;149:55–72.
15. Sarmiento A. The brachioradialis as a deforming force in Colles' fractures. Clin Orthop Relat Res. 1965;38:86–92.
16. Knirk JL, Jupiter JB. Intra-articular fractures of the distal end of the radius in young adults. J Bone Joint Surg Am. 1986;68(5):647–59.

17. Schumer ED, Leslie BM. Fragment-specific fixation of distal radius fractures using the Trimed device. Tech Hand Up Extrem Surg. 2005;9(2):74–83.
18. Lam J, Wolfe SW. Distal radius fractures: what cannot be fixed with a volar plate? The role of fragment-specific fixation in modern fracture treatment. Oper Tech Sports Med. 2010;18:181–8.
19. Iba K, Ozasa Y, Wada T, Kamiya T, Yamashita T, Aoki M. Efficacy of radial styloid targeting screws in volar plate fixation of intra-articular distal radial fractures: a biomechanical study in a cadaver fracture model. J Orthop Surg Res. 2010;5:90.
20. Wei DH, Raizman NM, Bottino CJ, Jobin CM, Strauch RJ, Rosenwasser MP. Unstable distal radial fractures treated with external fixation, a radial column plate, or a volar plate. A prospective randomized trial. J Bone Joint Surg Am. 2009;91(7):1568–77.
21. Singh S, Trikha P, Twyman R. Superficial radial nerve damage due to kirschner wiring of the radius. Injury. 2005;36(2):330–2.

Chapter 10
Distal Radius Fracture: Kapandji (Intrafocal) Pinning Technique

Andy Zhu, Jared Thomas, and Jeffrey N. Lawton

Case

The patient is a 60-year-old right hand dominant female who presented for evaluation of right wrist pain which began after she slipped on ice and landed on her outstretched right arm. Physical exam and X-ray of the right wrist revealed a dorsally displaced and angulated, closed distal radius fracture with intra-articular extension into the radiocarpal joint and DRUJ and significant loss of palmar tilt (Fig. 10.1a, b).

Sensation and motor function were intact to all nerve distributions. A hematoma block was administered and the fracture was reduced and placed in a sugar-tong splint. Post-reduction films demonstrated some residual dorsal angulation but overall improvement in palmar tilt (Fig. 10.1c, d). She presented to the Hand clinic 5 days later and after a detailed history and physical exam as well as review of the X-rays, surgical fixation was recommended.

A. Zhu, MD (✉) • J. Thomas, MD (✉) • J.N. Lawton, MD
Department of Orthopaedic Surgery, University of Michigan Health System, A. Alfred Taubman Health Care Center, Floor 2, Reception: B 2912 Taubman Center, 1500 East Medical Center Drive, Ann Arbor, MI 48109-5328, USA
e-mail: zandy@med.umich.edu; tjared@med.umich.edu

© Springer International Publishing Switzerland 2016   121
J.N. Lawton (ed.), *Distal Radius Fractures*,
DOI 10.1007/978-3-319-27489-8_10

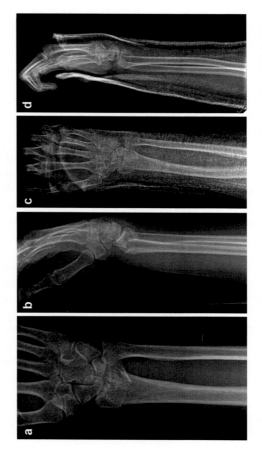

Fig. 10.1 (**a**, **b**) PA and lateral Injury films of Right Wrist. (**c**, **d**) PA and lateral post-reduction films of Right Wrist

Due to the patient's strong preference against open reduction internal fixation or external fixation, closed reduction and pinning was offered.

She was taken to the operating room 1 week after initial injury where closed reduction was performed under fluoroscopy. Once palmar tilt was restored beyond neutral and radial inclination restored with gentle traction and maneuvering, a single 0.045 in. Kirschner wire was inserted in retrograde fashion through the radial styloid engaging both the distal fragment and the metaphysis proximal to the fracture fragment. Two Kirschner wires were inserted dorsally into the fracture site by Kapandji technique and confirmed with fluoroscopy. The fracture was then manipulated using the two wires to restore palmar tilt. The wires were sequentially drilled engaging the volar cortex proximal to the fracture site holding the reduction (Fig. 10.2a, b). The pins were left outside the skin, cut, and bent. A well-padded sugar-tong splint was then placed.

Postoperatively the patient remained in the sugar-tong splint in supination for 2 weeks before transitioning to a short arm cast. Pins were removed 4 week postoperatively; and the patient remained immobilized in a short arm cast for a total of 6 weeks. After removal of the short arm cast at week 6 she was transitioned to a thermoplastic splint and encouraged to begin formal rehabilitation with occupational therapy emphasizing forearm, wrist, and digital range of motion. Three months postoperatively she returned to clinic and demonstrated full range of motion without any deficits.

History

Adalbert Kapandji was son of Mehmed Kapandji, a general surgeon most well known in Hand Surgery for his work with Louis Sauvé in the development of the Sauvé-Kapandji procedure for chronic dislocation of the distal radioulnar joint [1]. Aldalbert Kapandji first described the double intrafocal pinning technique in 1976 in the Annales De Chirurgie [2]. The goals of the procedure as outlined by Kapandji were the following: obtain a bone fusion

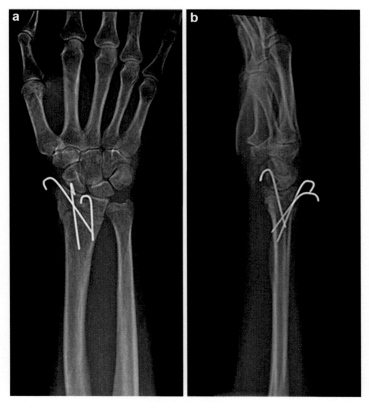

Fig. 10.2 (**a**, **b**) Postoperative PA and lateral wrist films

in good position by strict retention and prevention of secondary collapse, avoid plaster cast and enable immediate functional rehabilitation to minimize trophic complications, and perform treatment with a simple surgical method. The technique was first described for management of Colles' type fracture patterns; a low energy, extra-articular, and dorsally displaced distal radius fracture with minimal comminution. As discussed later in this chapter, indications have since expanded with good results.

Kapandji's original technique began with closed manual reduction to restore anatomic alignment of the fracture fragment (Fig. 10.3). While maintaining reduction, a radial to ulnar pin is introduced directly into the fracture site. The pin is advanced to the center of the fracture gap and elevated to provide a buttressing effect restoring radial inclination. The pin is then driven through the ulnar cortex of the radius securing fixation. This technique is then performed in similar fashion with a dorsal to volar pin directed at the volar cortex to restore volar tilt. Postoperatively, Kapandji advocated immediate wrist mobilization and avoidance of a plaster cast. Depending upon the patient, many do supplement with a fiberglass short arm cast.

Kapandji's two pin intrafocal technique gained widespread popularity in Europe following its description in 1976 with numerous publications reporting on this technique [3–7]. Early advocators of the technique adhered to Kapandji's original description with the use of two pins; however, as indications expanded modifications of the technique began to occur. Peyroux et al. reported on a case series of 159 patients with distal radius fractures treated with Kapandji intrafocal pinning. Their study advocated the use of a third dorsal medial pin in distal radius fractures with significant dorsal comminution [6]. In 1987 Kapandji published an article discussing his technique 10 years after its initial introduction. In this article he also described the use of a third dorsal to volar posteromedial pin for complicated fractures involving multiple fragments and/or with articular surface involvement [8].

Since the introduction of the intrafocal pinning technique many modifications of the procedure have appeared within the orthopedic literature. Most modifications incorporate the buttressing effect of intrafocal pinning and augment this fixation with additional stabilization methods. Modifications have ranged from intrafocal intramedullary pinning [9] to combined static and intrafocal pinning [10] to intrafocal pinning with plate stabilization [11]. The use of Kapandji pinning has not only been limited to dorsally displaced distal radius fractures as it has also been described for treatment of anterior displaced fractures. In 1995 Hoël and Kapandji described two additional anterior approaches to his intrafocal pinning technique to address volar displaced fractures [12].

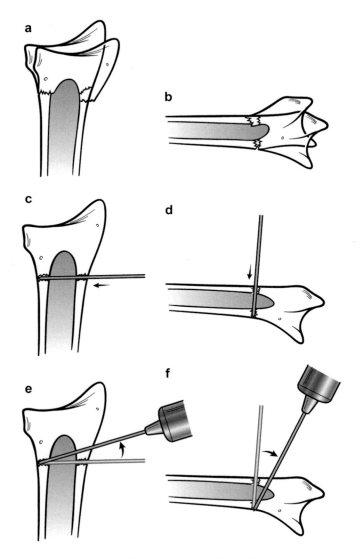

Fig. 10.3 Kapandji original two pin intrafocal technique. (**a**, **b**) Angulated fracture in PA and lateral projections. (**c**, **d**) Placement of K-wire through fracture to engage volar cortex. (**e**, **f**) Manipulation of K-wire, distally, to improve alignment and reduce fracture

Indications

Kapandji's technique was originally indicated for displaced, extra-articular Colles' fractures with minimal posterior comminution in young patients with good bone stock. Colles' originally description of the fracture pattern included a "depression" of the "posterior surface" of the arm with the ulna "projecting towards the palm and inner edge of the limb" [13]. Colles' fractures are presently described as a distal radius fracture with dorsal comminution, dorsal angulation, dorsal displacement, radial shortening, and associated fracture of the ulna styloid [14]. Early case series of intrafocal pinning of distal radius fractures focused on extra-articular Colles' fractures with minimal to moderate dorsal cortex comminution [3]. At that time, a simple three stage classification was commonly applied to describe the amount of comminution on the dorsal aspect of the fracture site. Currently, the most common classifications of distal radius fractures include the Frykman, Mayo, Melone, and AO/OT. Variable interobserver and intraobserver reliability have made these classification systems difficult to apply with little value with regards to optimal management [15].

The basic principle of intrafocal pinning is to create a buttress effect on a displaced distal fragment thus preventing subsequent collapse and allowing for anatomic healing. This is most readily achieved in fractures with a large fragment, minimal comminution, and good quality bone. Articular involvement, multiple fragments, and comminution do not preclude the use of intrafocal pinning as long as adequate reduction can be maintained. Irreducible fractures are not amendable to pinning and require direct visualization and reduction. Classically described for dorsal angulated and displaced fractures, this technique has also been applied in volar angulated and displaced (Smith's) fractures as well [12, 16]. One must obviously be cognizant of the relevant local anatomy including the Radial Artery, Palmar Cutaneous Branch, and the Median Nerve, however.

The Kapandji intrafocal pinning has traditionally been performed in the adult population; however, its use has also been recently documented in the pediatric population [17, 18]. The pediatric population has great remodeling potential and does not necessitate surgical fixation for distal radius fractures with minimal displacement and angulation. Dorsal and/or radial angulation more than 30° after age 8, more than 20° after age 10, and more than 15° after age 13 may benefit from intrafocal pinning [17].

Currently the AAOS clinical practice guideline summary recommends surgical fixation for distal radius fractures with postreduction radial shortening >3 mm, dorsal tilt >10°, or intra-articular displacement or step-off >2 mm as opposed to cast fixation. They are unable to recommend for or against any one specific surgical method for fixation of distal radius fractures [19]. At our institution ORIF with volar plating is still the most common method of fixation; however, we have experienced good results with use of the intrafocal pinning technique when performed for select fractures.

Technique

The operation can be performed under general or regional anesthesia. A tourniquet should be placed over the arm at the surgeon's discretion. First, the fracture is reduced under fluoroscopic guidance. Finger traps may be used before or during the case with 5–10 lbs of counter traction applied to aid in reduction. The goal of the reduction is to restore radial height while recreating anatomic radial inclination and volar tilt. Often one hand can be used to maintain reduction and allow for fracture manipulation while the other hand directs fixation.

The order and number of Kirschner wires inserted will depend on multiple factors including: technique, fracture pattern, and quality of bone. The original technique described by Kapandji begins with a lateral Kirschner wire. A number of wire sizes can be used. We typically prefer 0.045 in. Kirschner wires. The wire is mounted on a wire driver and directed in-line with the fracture gap. Prior to insertion a small cutaneous incision is made and dissected bluntly down to bone to avoid injury to the sensory branches of the radial nerve as well as the extensor tendons. The wire is inserted into the center of the fracture gap. The drill is then raised 45° or until the wire buttresses the proximal fragment restoring radial inclination. The wire is then passed through the far cortex securing the fixation. Kapandji's original description then involved insertion of a dorsal to volar wire in a similar fashion with the starting point centered about the third metacarpal axis. It is important to evaluate the amount and location of the dorsal comminution in order to place a wire that can support areas of comminution. Common entry points include between the second and third extensor compartments and the fourth and fifth extensor compartments. The wire is again driven into the fracture gap, levered distally, and driven into the far volar cortex. If two dorsal to volar wires are to be used, then both wires are first introduced into the fracture gap. The wires are simultaneously levered distally to improve palmar tilt, then driven into the far cortex. Modifications of the technique include placements of static wires, anterior to posterior directed wires, external fixation, and plate fixation.

After pin insertion, fluoroscopy is used to evaluate alignment and stability. Passive finger and wrist flexion is examined to ensure no tendons have been tethered. Any skin tethering is released with a blade. Pins can be cut and left buried or bent and cut approximately 1 cm from the skin. Caps may be placed over pins left outside the skin. A well-padded sugar-tong splint is placed postoperatively. Pins are removed approximately 4 weeks postoperatively. The patient typically is transitioned from a splint to a short arm cast after 1 week. The patient remains in a cast for approximately 6 weeks and transitioned into a removable splint at which time formal occupational therapy and/or home therapy is initiated. Alternatively, a removable splint may be employed early on as described by Kapandji.

Tips/Tricks

- A stack of towels placed under wrist allows for true lateral fluoroscopic shots to guide pin placement without significant wrist motion or disturbance of fracture reduction
- Additional pins should be used as needed to ensure a stable construct and avoid dorsal collapse
- Additional pins can be used as appropriate as joysticks to reduce and provide fixation to individual fracture fragments based upon the complexity of the comminution

Kapandji advocated immediate wrist mobilization without a plaster cast as one of his primary goals of percutaneous pinning. Immediate mobilization was initially widely practiced; however, currently common practice is to provide a period of immobilization postoperatively—obviously, this depends upon one's comfort with patient reliability.

Results

While Kapandji's original manuscript provided a detailed description of the procedure, very little information was reported regarding results. Epinette et al. [3] were one of the first groups to publish their study on 72 cases. The majority of the fractures were extra-articular Colles' type fractures; however, they did expand the originally described indications to include intra-articular fractures and fractures of elderly patients. They performed the original two pin technique and placed the extremity in a sling without plaster casting postoperatively. Complications were associated with 26 % of patients including secondary displacement (5), tendon injuries (5), and pain and swelling syndromes (6). Only 7 % of patients experienced a negative final result related to these complications. Their results demonstrated that 93 % of operated wrists were pain free, 80 % regained full grip strength, and an overall 84 % good and excellent results. Peyroux et al. [6] treated 159 cases of distal radius fractures with the Kapandji technique and introduced the use of a third pin for more complex fracture patterns. However, the majority of the fractures were extra-articular fractures with minimal to moderate posterior comminution. Postoperatively plaster casts were placed for any fixation that demonstrated movement at the fracture gap with flexion and extension. Complications included secondary displacement (10), infection (2), pin migration (7), tendinous complications (4), and nervous complications (2). Results revealed 91 % subjective good/very good results, 93 % good/very good range of motion, and 73 % good/very good radiographic results. Subsequent large scale studies expanded indications and also demonstrated more frequent use of plaster casting all with largely satisfactory results [7, 20].

The three pin technique was reported in the North American orthopedic literature by Greatings et al. [21]. They retrospectively reviewed 23 patients treated with three pin Kapandji technique and short arm casting. They reported 7 excellent, 4 good, and 2 fair clinical results. Fritz et al. [10] introduced the concept of static and dynamic combinational pinning. They described fracture reduction through the original Kapandji technique with subsequent insertion of 1 to 2 static K-wires. They analyzed 110 fractures with 35 % excellent, 50 % good, 10 % fair, and 5 % poor results according to NYOH scores. They had a 23 % complication rate with the most frequent involving paresthesia in the area of the superficial radial nerve. Strohm et al. [22] performed a randomized trial of traditional static pinning described by Willenegger and Guggenbuhl [23] compared to the modified Kapandji described by Fritz et al. [10]. One hundred consecutive patients with Colles' fractures were treated with the same postoperative standardized care. Martini score for patients treated with the modified Kapandji method was on average good to very good compared to satisfactory to good for patients treated with the Willenegger technique.

Handol et al. performed a Cochrane review on percutaneous pinning of distal radius fractures and concluded that while there was some evidence to support the use of percutaneous pinning, no recommendation could be made on type and indications for pinning [24]. It was noted that Kapadnji type pinning was found to have higher risks of complications in trials included in the review. Common complications associated with Kapandji pinning include loss of fracture reduction, tendon rupture, radial sensory nerve irritation, and reflex sympathetic dystrophy (Table 10.1).

There have been recent publications of the use Kapandji technique in the pediatric population for distal radius fractures with severe deformity. Parikh et al. performed a retrospective case review comparing 10 cases of intrafocal pinning to 26 cases of conventional pinning for dorsally angulated metaphyseal distal radius fracture with an open distal radial physis [17]. Both groups achieved union with pain-free range of motion. There was no statistical significance between complications of the two groups. Satish et al. treated 46 children between the age of 7–14 years old with Kapandji intrafocal technique with extrafocal wire augmentation

Table 10.1 Complications of kapandji pinning technique

Complications
Fracture displacement
Tendon injuries
Tethering
Rupture
Nerve injury
Superficial radial nerve
Carpal tunnel syndrome
Infections
Pin site
Wound
CRPS

for displaced, closed, non-physeal distal radius fractures [18]. Near anatomic reduction was achieved in all cases with complete union and full range of motion restored.

References

1. Sebastin SJ, Larson BP, Chung KC. History and evolution of the Sauve-Kapandji procedure. J Hand Surg Am. 2012;37(9):1895–902.
2. Kapandji A. Internal fixation by double intrafocal plate. Functional treatment of non articular fractures of the lower end of the radius (author's transl). Ann Chir. 1976;30(11–12):903–8.
3. Epinette JA, Lehut JM, Cavenaile M, Bouretz JC, Decoulx J. Pouteau-Colles fracture: double-closed "basket-like" pinning according to Kapandji. Apropos of a homogeneous series of 70 cases. Ann Chir Main. 1982;1(1): 71–83.
4. Docquier J, Soete P, Twahirwa J, Flament A. Kapandji's method of intra-focal nailing in Pouteau-Colles fractures. Acta Orthop Belg. 1982;48(5): 794–810.
5. Kerboul B, Le Saout J, Lefevre C, Miroux D, Fabre L, Le Noac'h JF, et al. Comparative study of 3 therapeutic methods for Pouteau Colles' fracture. Apropos of 97 cases. J Chir (Paris). 1986;123(6–7):428–34.

6. Peyroux LM, Dunaud JL, Caron M, Ben Slamia I, Kharrat M. The Kapandji technique and its evolution in the treatment of fractures of the distal end of the radius. Report on a series of 159 cases. Ann Chir Main. 1987;6(2): 109–22.

7. Nonnenmacher J, Kempf I. Role of intrafocal pinning in the treatment of wrist fractures. Int Orthop. 1988;12(2):155–62.

8. Kapandji A. Intra-focal pinning of fractures of the distal end of the radius 10 years later. Ann Chir Main. 1987;6(1):57–63.

9. Walton NP, Brammar TJ, Hutchinson J, Raj D, Coleman NP. Treatment of unstable distal radial fractures by intrafocal, intramedullary K-wires. Injury. 2001;32(5):383–9.

10. Fritz T, Wersching D, Klavora R, Krieglstein C, Friedl W. Combined Kirschner wire fixation in the treatment of Colles fracture. A prospective, controlled trial. Arch Orthop Trauma Surg. 1999;119(3–4):171–8.

11. Nonnenmacher J, Soley K, Bahm J. Intrafocal wire fixation of wrist fractures. The original Kapandji technique. Course. Review of 400 cases. Chirurgie. 1994;120(3):119–27.

12. Hoel G, Kapandji AI. Osteosynthesis using intra-focal pins of anteriorly dislocated fractures of the inferior radial epiphysis. Ann Chir Main Memb Super. 1995;14(3):142–56. discussion 156–7.

13. Colles A. On the fracture of the carpal extremity of the radius. Edinb Med Surg J. 1814;10:181. Clin Orthop Relat Res. 2006;445:5–7.

14. Green DP, Wolfe SW. Green's operative hand surgery. Philadelphia: Saunders/Elsevier; 2011. p. 2 v. (xvi, 2240, I–60 p).

15. Kural C, Sungur I, Kaya I, Ugras A, Erturk A, Cetinus E. Evaluation of the reliability of classification systems used for distal radius fractures. Orthopedics. 2010;33(11):801.

16. Guichet JM, Moller CC, Dautel G, Lascombes P. A modified Kapandji procedure for Smith's fracture in children. J Bone Joint Surg Br. 1997;79(5): 734–7.

17. Parikh SN, Jain VV, Youngquist J. Intrafocal pinning for distal radius metaphyseal fractures in children. Orthopedics. 2013;36(6):783–8.

18. Satish BR, Vinodkumar M, Suresh M, Seetharam PY, Jaikumar K. Closed reduction and K-wiring with the Kapandji technique for completely displaced pediatric distal radial fractures. Orthopedics. 2014;37(9):e810–6.

19. Lichtman DM, Bindra RR, Boyer MI, Putnam MD, Ring D, Slutsky DJ, et al. Treatment of distal radius fractures. J Am Acad Orthop Surg. 2010;18(3):180–9.

20. Nonnenmacher J, Neumeier K. Intrafocal wiring of fractures of the wrist joint. Handchir Mikrochir Plast Chir. 1987;19(2):67–70.

21. Greatting MD, Bishop AT. Intrafocal (Kapandji) pinning of unstable fractures of the distal radius. Orthop Clin North Am. 1993;24(2):301–7.

22. Strohm PC, Muller CA, Boll T, Pfister U. Two procedures for Kirschner wire osteosynthesis of distal radial fractures. A randomized trial. J Bone Joint Surg Am. 2004;86-A(12):2621–8.

23. Willenegger H, Guggenbuhl A. Operative treatment of certain cases of distal radius fracture. Helv Chir Acta. 1959;26(2):81–94.
24. Handoll HH, Vaghela MV, Madhok R. Percutaneous pinning for treating distal radial fractures in adults. Cochrane Database Syst Rev. 2007;3, CD006080.

Chapter 11
Bridge Plating for Distal Radius Fractures

Mark C. Shreve and Kevin J. Malone

Case Presentation

A 37-year-old right-hand dominant morbidly obese female with a past medical history of obstructive sleep apnea and asthma was involved in a motor vehicle accident. She sustained a right open tibial shaft fracture, a manubrium fracture with a retrosternal hematoma and a left closed distal radius fracture (Fig. 11.1). She presented with numbness and tingling in the median nerve distribution which improved with closed reduction of the radius fracture. Upon taking her history, she was found to have pre-injury symptoms consistent with carpal tunnel syndrome. On admission to the Level 1 trauma center she underwent irrigation, debridement,

M.C. Shreve, MD (✉)
The CORE Institute, 26750 Providence Parkway, Suite 200, Novi, MI 48374, USA
e-mail: Mark.Shreve@thecoreinstitute.com

K.J. Malone, MD
Department of Orthopaedic Surgery, University Hospitals Case Medical Center, 11100 Euclid Avenue, Cleveland, OH 44106, USA

© Springer International Publishing Switzerland 2016
J.N. Lawton (ed.), *Distal Radius Fractures*,
DOI 10.1007/978-3-319-27489-8_11

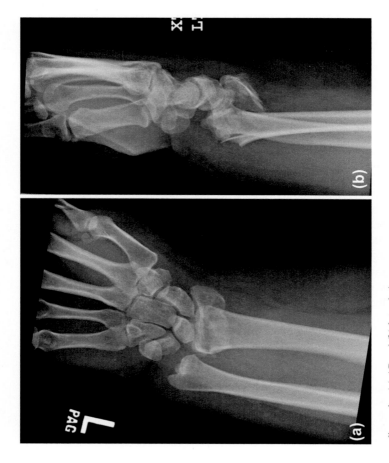

Fig. 11.1 Injury radiographs. (**a**) AP and (**b**) lateral views

and intramedullary nailing of the open tibia fracture with reduction and splinting of her distal radius fracture. The next day she returned to the operating room for definitive fixation of the distal radius fracture. Given her lower extremity injury and the need for immediate weight bearing on the upper extremities for early mobilization she underwent open reduction and internal fixation of the distal radius fracture with a dorsal spanning bridge plate with supplemental radial styloid Kirschner wire fixation (Fig. 11.2). After fixation of the radius fracture she underwent an open carpal tunnel release. The distal radioulnar joint was tested for stability and was found to be stable; and she was then placed in a sugar-tong splint in slight supination. She was allowed to immediately weight bear on the injured extremity through the forearm for transfers and mobilization. Twelve weeks later, after the radius fracture had healed on radiographs, she returned to the operating room, and the dorsal bridge plate and the Kirschner wire were removed. (Figs. 11.3 and 11.4) She was placed into a soft dressing and was not restricted postoperatively.

Introduction

Distal radius fractures are commonly encountered fractures, accounting for one sixth of all fractures treated in emergency rooms in the United States [1, 2]. Not all distal radius fractures, in terms of fracture anatomy and patient characteristics, are amenable to solely volar locked plating that has become the mainstay of treatment. Burke and Singer first described the technique of dorsal distraction plating for highly comminuted distal radius fractures in 1998 [3]. In some situations this technique can be quite useful for stabilizing and reducing certain fractures, relying on the method of ligamentotaxis to aid in obtaining and maintaining reduction, and serving as a dorsal buttress for the comminuted fracture fragments. Also known as internal bridge plating, the technique has proven useful in high-energy comminuted distal radius fractures with metaphyseal and diaphyseal extension [4], in polytrauma patients with concomitant lower extremity or pelvic fractures [5], in elderly

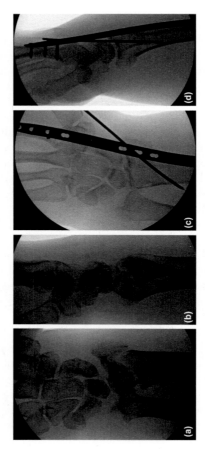

Fig. 11.2 Intra-operative fluoroscopy views. (**a**) Traction AP, (**b**) traction lateral, (**c**) AP, and (**d**) lateral

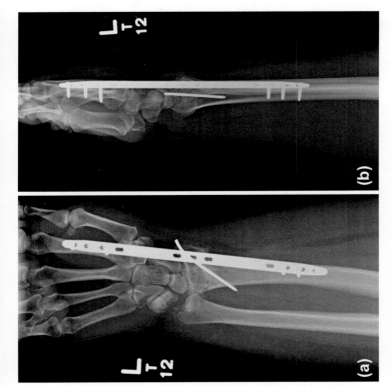

Fig. 11.3 Radiographs at 2 months postoperatively. (**a**) AP and (**b**) lateral views

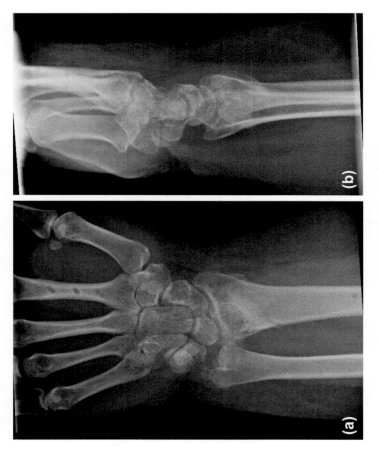

Fig. 11.4 Radiographs at 4 months postoperatively after plate removal. (**a**) AP and (**b**) lateral views

patients with potentially poor bone quality [6], and even in the salvage of distal radius nonunions [7]. While many of these situations may have previously been treated with external fixation, bridge plating has the benefit of an all internal design.

Review of the Literature

The technique of bridge plating for distal radius fractures was first described by Burke and Singer in the late 1990s [3]. They discussed opening the wrist dorsally through the 4th compartment and using a 9-hole 3.5 mm dynamic compression plate secured distally to the 3rd metacarpal shaft and proximally to the radial shaft. Their indications were for any displaced and comminuted distal radius fracture and excluded extraarticular and volar shear pattern injuries. Additional Kirschner wire fixation was used for displaced articular fragments. They routinely removed the plate at 8–10 weeks postoperatively. No cases of reflex sympathetic dystrophy were reported, however no outcomes data on any of their cases were discussed, only providing one case report.

An alternative technique of internal distraction plating was described by Becton et al., with distal fixation on the index metacarpal instead of the 3rd metacarpal [8]. The plate was placed in the floor of the 2nd dorsal compartment as opposed to the 4th dorsal compartment in Burke and Singer's technique. During early use of the procedure they performed a wide dorsal approach, but later changed to making two smaller incision, one distally over the index metacarpal and one proximally over the radial shaft, sliding the plate retrograde through the compartment. They used a specially made 3.5 mm dorsal bridge plate from Biomet (Warsaw, IN). They reported their results of 35 cases, although from six different surgeons, and found no cases of reflex sympathetic dystrophy. Two complications were reported, one patient with an index metacarpal fracture through a screw hole and one patient with loosening of the index metacarpal screws. Both patients ultimately healed their radius fractures.

Noting a complication rate upwards of 62 % [9] when using an external fixation device for treating comminuted and displaced distal radius fractures, Chhabra et al. [10] performed a biomechanical comparison of the internal distraction plating and external fixation. Using an acrylic rod model to simulate an unstable distal radius fracture, they compared two commercially available metal plates used as an internal bridge plate, and three external fixator devices commonly used. Results showed that the internal fixator plates were more rigid than the external fixation devices in axial compression. The internal fixator devices showed significantly greater stiffness in tension, compression, and lateral bending, however in anteroposterior bending the external fixation devices were stiffer. They concluded that using an internal fixation device would help prevent dorsal collapse and function better as a rigid dorsal buttress.

With higher energy distal radius fractures having metaphyseal and diaphyseal comminution, treatment with bridging external fixation may not provide adequate stability proximal to the metaphysis [4]. Seeing this as an issue, Ruch and colleagues utilized the technique for treatment of distal radius fractures in this clinical situation and reported good overall results in 22 patients [4]. They secured the plate distally to the third metacarpal, using a three incision technique, with the third incision centered over Lister's tubercle. This third incision provided direct access to the metaphysis to place bone graft or add supplemental fixation. Bone graft was used in 11 patients in their study. The plates were removed at an average of 124 days postoperatively. At final follow-up, flexion and extension averaged 57° and 65°, respectively, and pronation and supination averaged 77° and 76°, respectively. They found that average DASH scores were 34 points at 6 months, 15 points at 1 year, and 11.5 points at final follow-up. These results highlighted that prolonged immobilization with the internal distraction plate resulted in a functional range of motion after removal and with minimal disability at final follow-up. Poly-traumatized patients were able to immediately weight bear for transfers and mobility and also were able to return to work with hardware in place.

In a review of their cohort of patients, Hanel et al. discussed the two patient populations that primarily benefit from the technique of internal distal radius bridge plating: those with high-energy fractures with metaphyseal and diaphyseal extension and those multiply injured patients requiring immediate weight bearing on the injured limb for early mobilization [5]. They treated 62 patients with a distal radius bridge plate secured to the index metacarpal shaft, first using a 22-hole 2.4 mm mandibular reconstruction plate (Synthes, Paoli, PA) and later using a specifically designed 20-hole 2.4 mm distal radius bridge plate from Synthes. Plates were removed at an average of 112 days. Return of functional range of motion occurred by 1 year and fracture healing occurred in all cases with no articular step-offs greater than 2 mm or distal radio-ulnar joint instability. They had no instances of excessive postoperative finger stiffness or reflex sympathetic dystrophy. One patient did have a ruptured extensor carpi radialis brevis (ECRB), but this patient had a fractured implant at 16 months postoperatively causing the rupture as he had failed to agree to removal due to occupational pressures.

In order to determine the necessary number of screws proximally and distally, Wolf et al. examined the construct in a cadaveric model of distal radius fractures [11]. Comparing the distal radius bridge plating technique to an external fixation system in axial load in flexion or extension, the authors found that the radiocarpal spanning 2.4 mm locking plate was significantly more stable than the external fixator. They found that only three locking screws were needed distally and three locking screws proximally.

Richard and colleagues examined the outcomes of internal distraction plating in older individuals with comminuted distal radius fractures, specifically those over 60 years old [6]. Using both the surgical technique by Ruch et al. [4] and Hanel et al. [5], they retrospectively reviewed 33 patients over 60 years of age, with an average age of 70 years. At a final follow-up (average 47 weeks) all fractures had healed and radiographs showed an average palmar tilt of 5° and average positive ulnar variance of 0.6 mm. Mean values for wrist flexion and extension were 46° and 50°, respectively, with supination and pronation 79° and 77°, respectively. Final mean DASH scores were 32. They noted 10 of 33 patients with digital stiffness with one requiring tenolysis, and one patient with complex regional pain syndrome.

Recently, Mithani et al. described using the spanning dorsal distraction plate technique in the salvage of distal radius nonunions [7]. They described utilizing the dorsal bridge plate either alone or in conjunction with non-spanning fixation, in 8 patients. All patients went on to union, with plate removal at an average of 148 days, with statistically significant improvements in arc of motion, supination, and DASH scores at final follow-up. One patient experienced persistent pain and ultimately required wrist arthrodesis.

Rationale for Approach

The presented patient was a morbidly obese young adult poly-trauma with a concomitant lower extremity injury. This injury precluded her from full weight bearing on the lower extremity necessitating early mobilization with an assistive device. Therefore it was important to perform an operation that could allow her to weight bear through the forearm early, and without exposed pins, which would be a potential nidus for infection given the likely prolonged stay in the intensive care unit. The internal distal radius bridge plating technique of fixation is a helpful alternative for quickly stabilizing and definitively treating the distal radius fracture that would allow the patient to immediately weight bear and use the extremity early in the post-injury course.

The indications for utilizing the distal radius bridge plating technique include:

- Patients with high-energy intraarticular distal radius fracture with metaphyseal and diaphyseal extension.
- Polytrauma patients with concomitant lower extremity or pelvic wounds to allow early mobilization assistance through the injured extremity.
- Elderly patients with intraarticular distal radius fracture with osteoporotic bone in which rigid fixation might not be achievable.
- Radiocarpal dislocation to provide stability as an alternative to external fixation or cast immobilization.
- As an adjunct for salvage of distal radial malunions.

Contraindications for the use of distal radius bridge plating include general contraindications to surgery, such as poor patient clinical status or active infection, and specifically any concomitant index or middle metacarpal shaft fractures.

Surgical Technique

The patient is placed supine on the operating table with an attached radiolucent hand table on the operative side. A well-padded tourniquet is placed on the upper arm and the arm is prepped and draped. Either a large or mini fluoroscopy machine may be utilized as desired. The arm is abducted at the shoulder onto the arm board and the Agee reduction maneuver is performed as described by Hanel et al. [5]. Longitudinal traction is applied to the distal radius by pulling distally on the index and middle fingers to bring the distal radius out to appropriate length. A palmarly directed translational force is applied to the carpus to reduce the dorsal subluxation and a pronation force is applied to the carpus to bring the carpus out of the usual supination deformity. Adequate articular reduction is confirmed under fluoroscopy. Sterile finger traps can then be placed on the index and middle fingers and attached to a sterile rope, which is then suspended from the end of the hand table with 10 lbs of weight to provide continuous longitudinal traction with the hand in pronation.

Prior to placement of the bridge plate, provisional fixation can also be obtained by placing a Kirschner wire, 1.6 or 2.0 mm, from the radial styloid into the proximal medial shaft of the distal radius. This can be done percutaneously or by making a longitudinal incision on the radial aspect of the wrist, distal to the radial styloid, and identifying the radial sensory nerve branches at this level. Placement of the Kirschner wire is confirmed under fluoroscopy.

We prefer to use the 2.4 mm distal radius bridge plate specifically designed for the bridge plating technique by Synthes (Paoli, PA) which allows placement of locking and non-locking screws proximally and distally, and has tapered ends to aid in sliding the plate within the 2nd extensor compartment. However, others have used

12- to 16-hole 3.5 mm dynamic compression plates [3, 4]. The larger plates need to be placed on the 3rd metacarpal and proximally through the 4th compartment oftentimes through an open technique whereas the smaller tapered plates can be placed distally on the 2nd metacarpal shaft and slid proximally through the floor of the 2nd compartment. The tapered plate is then placed over the skin and fluoroscopic imaging is used to confirm proper placement over the 2nd metacarpal shaft and the radial shaft, and this can be marked on the skin. A 4 cm incision is then made at the base of the 2nd metacarpal. Any radial sensory nerve branches are identified and gently retracted and protected. The insertion of the extensor carpi radialis longus (ECRL) and ECRB is identified at the base of the 2nd and 3rd metacarpals, respectively. A second incision of about 4 to 5 cm is made at the proximal extent of the planned plate insertion over the radial shaft, just proximal to the outcropper muscles (extensor pollicis brevis and abductor pollicis longus) and in line with the ECRL and ECRB muscle bellies. The interval between these muscles is developed revealing the underlying radial shaft.

The distal radius bridge plate is then inserted, starting in the proximal incision, between the ECRL and ECRB muscles in the floor of the 2nd compartment from proximal to distal until it is visualized in the distal incision base. The plate rests extraperiosteally and within the 2nd dorsal compartment. If the plate is unable to be passed distally, a suture passer or guide wire can be passed retrograde through the 2nd compartment and then fixed to the distal end of the plate and used to guide it to the distal incision. Also a third incision can be made over Lister's tubercle and the 2nd compartment opened to pass the plate under direct visualization.

The plate position is then confirmed fluoroscopically to be centered over the index metacarpal shaft and radial shaft. Then a 2.7 mm non-locking cortical screw is placed through the most distal hole of the plate into the index metacarpal. It is imperative to ensure that this is exactly in the center of the bone so as not to produce a rotational malalignment of the hand relative to the radial shaft. Also note that this first screw placed is a non-locking screw, so as to pull the plate securely to the bone. The traction is then removed from the wrist prior to placing a screw in the most proximal aspect of the plate, so as to avoid over-distraction of the radiocarpal joint. Another 2.7 mm cortical non-locking screw is then placed in the most proximal hole in the radial shaft to also lag the plate to the bone. Then two 2.7 mm locking screws are placed in the plate proximally, as well as two more 2.7 mm locking screws placed in the plate distally. This gives a minimum of three screws at either end of the plate.

Depending upon the fracture configuration, a third dorsal incision centered over Lister's tubercle, if previously made, can be used to reduce any remaining malreduced articular fragments or for placement of metaphyseal bone graft if necessary. The three holes in the middle section of the plate, overlying the distal radius metaphysis, can be used to lag any free metaphyseal or articular cortical pieces if desired. Fluoroscopy is then used to confirm adequate and satisfactory reduction. Any Kirschner wires placed are then cut to be buried below the skin. The wounds are then irrigated with sterile saline and closed in layers in an interrupted fashion using absorbable sutures for the subcutaneous tissues and non-absorbable sutures for the skin.

The stability of the distal radioulnar joint (DRUJ) is then assessed in pronation and supination. If the DRUJ is stable, then the patient is splinted in slight supination using a sugar-tong splint for the first 2 weeks. If the DRUJ is unstable, then the ulnar head can be reduced into the sigmoid notch and two 1.6 mm Kirschner wires can be placed transversely from the ulna into the radius just proximal to the DRUJ or the triangular fibrocartilage complex can be repaired by open means.

The patient is allowed to weight bear through the forearm immediately using a platform walker or crutches. Occupational therapy can also begin digital range of motion exercises shortly after surgery.

Supplemental Kirschner wire fixation can be typically removed at 6 weeks postoperatively. The distal radius bridge plate is removed no earlier than 12 weeks after surgery once the fracture has healed. Removal can be performed as an outpatient procedure under local or regional anesthesia. The previous incisions are opened and the screws are removed. The plate is then slid distally through the distal incision. No immobilization is used after plate removal, just a soft, padded dressing.

Tips/tricks

- Avoid placing the plate too distal on the index metacarpal. After plate fixation check to ensure there is full passive flexion of the fingers to avoid postoperative digital stiffness.
- Ensure that the plate is placed in the center of the metacarpal shaft so as to prevent any rotary displacement of the hand relative to the radial shaft.
- Reduction of the distal radius fracture is best performed with longitudinal traction, palmar translation, and pronation. Avoid direct pressure on the carpal tunnel. Perform carpal tunnel release when clinically necessary in the appropriate patients.
- Avoid over-distraction of the radiocarpal joint as this can limit postoperative digital motion and have an increased risk of the development of complex regional pain syndrome. Release the longitudinal traction weight prior to fixation proximally on the radial shaft to help prevent over-distraction.
- Do not hesitate to provide supplemental Kirschner wire fixation or apply bone graft when clinically relevant.

References

1. Court-Brown CM, Caesar B. Epidemiology of adult fractures: a review. Injury. 2006;37:691–7.
2. Graff S, Jupiter J. Fracture of the distal radius: classification of treatment and indications for external fixation. Injury. 1994;25 Suppl 4:S-D14-25.
3. Burke EF, Singer RM. Treatment of comminuted distal radius with the use of an internal distraction plate. Tech Hand Up Extrem Surg. 1998;2:248–52.
4. Ruch DS, Ginn TA, Yang CC, Smith BP, Rushing J, Hanel DP. Use of a distraction plate for distal radial fractures with metaphyseal and diaphyseal comminution. J Bone Joint Surg Am. 2005;87:945–54.
5. Hanel DP, Lu TS, Weil WM. Bridge plating of distal radius fractures: the Harborview method. Clin Orthop Relat Res. 2006;445:91–9.
6. Richard MJ, Katolik LI, Hanel DP, Wartinbee DA, Ruch DS. Distraction plating for the treatment of highly comminuted distal radius fractures in elderly patients. J Hand Surg Am. 2012;37:948–56.
7. Mithani SK, Srinivasan RC, Kamal R, Richard MJ, Leversedge FJ, Ruch DS. Salvage of distal radius nonunion with a dorsal spanning distraction plate. J Hand Surg Am. 2014;39:981–4.

8. Becton JL, Colborn GL, Goodrich JA. Use of an internal fixator device to treat comminuted fractures of the distal radius: report of a technique. Am J Orthop (Belle Mead NJ). 1998;27:619–23.

9. Weber SC, Szabo RM. Severely comminuted distal radial fracture as an unsolved problem: complications associated with external fixation and pins and plaster techniques. J Hand Surg Am. 1986;11:157–65.

10. Chhabra A, Hale JE, Milbrandt TA, Carmines DV, Degnan GG. Biomechanical efficacy of an internal fixator for treatment of distal radius fractures. Clin Orthop Relat Res. 2001;393:318–25.

11. Wolf JC, Weil WM, Hanel DP, Trumble TE. A biomechanic comparison of an internal radiocarpal-spanning 2.4-mm locking plate and external fixation in a model of distal radius fractures. J Hand Surg Am. 2006;31:1578–86.

Chapter 12
External Fixation and Percutaneous Pinning for Distal Radius Fractures

Laura W. Lewallen and Marco Rizzo

Case Presentation

A 48-year-old female fell onto her outstretched hand and sustained an injury to her right wrist. She was otherwise healthy and her past medical history was negative for prior fracture or any medical issues. On presentation, she displayed significant swelling and limited motion secondary to pain. She had gross deformity of the wrist. The skin was intact and she denied fingertip numbness and tingling.

Physical Assessment

Physical exam demonstrated significant tenderness about the distal radius. There was no elbow pain or tenderness. The fingers had some swelling, but no tenderness to palpation. Digital motion was limited secondary to pain. The skin was intact. She had normal sensation and capillary refill of the digits.

L.W. Lewallen, MD • M. Rizzo, MD (✉)
Department of Orthopedic Surgery, Mayo Clinic,
200 1st St SW, Rochester, MN 55905, USA
e-mail: lewallen.laura@mayo.edu; rizzo.marco@mayo.edu

© Springer International Publishing Switzerland 2016   151
J.N. Lawton (ed.), *Distal Radius Fractures*,
DOI 10.1007/978-3-319-27489-8_12

Diagnostic Studies and Diagnosis

Anteroposterior (AP) and lateral radiographs (Fig. 12.1a, b) demonstrated a displaced and dorsally angulated distal radius fracture. Significant shortening of the radius was appreciated on the AP view. In addition, the radial inclination was diminished. The fracture appeared to be intra-articular but with minimal step-off along the radiocarpal joint.

Management Options

Treatment options for this injury include both non-operative and operative intervention. The fracture pattern is such that most would agree that reduction is necessary. The primary consideration would be to perform a closed reduction in the acute setting. This was in fact performed. However, adequate maintenance of the reduction was impossible following splinting. Therefore discussion regarding surgery to maintain the reduction ensued. Different methods of fixation could be considered including open reduction and internal fixation using either a volar locking plate, fragment specific fixation or dorsal plate. In addition, one could consider spanning the fracture with a dorsal spanning plate. Finally, closed reduction and pinning with application of an external fixator was another option.

Management Chosen (Fig. 12.2a, b)

After careful deliberation and discussion of all surgical options with the patient, the latter was performed. She was taken to the operating room after undergoing regional anesthesia. The extremity underwent sterile prepping and was draped to expose the arm, wrist, and hand. Fluoroscopy was used to help visualize reduction and hardware placement. The index and long fingers were placed into sterile finger-traps to allow for 10–15 lbs of traction. The fracture was then manipulated to correct dorsal tilt and realign the

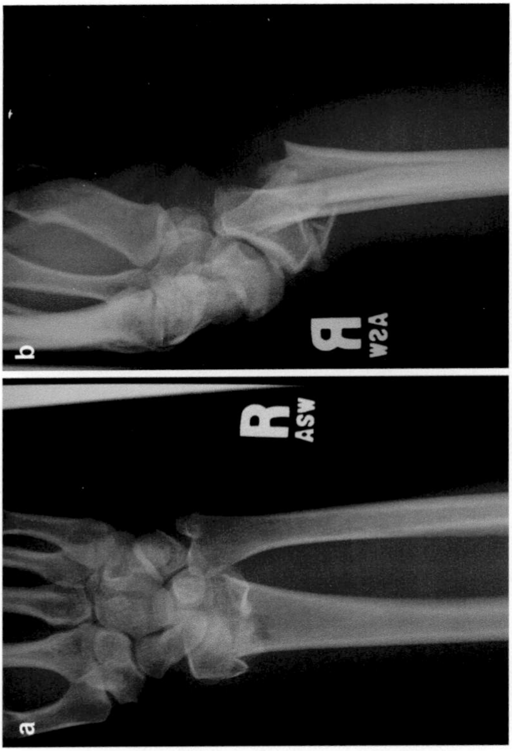

Fig. 12.1 A 48-year-old right hand-dominant female sustained an injury to her right wrist following a fall onto her outstretched hand. (**a**) PA and (**b**) lateral films demonstrate intra-articular distal radius fracture with dorsal angulation

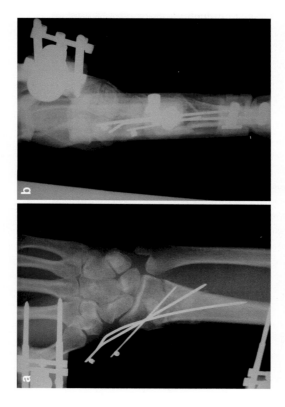

Fig. 12.2 (a) PA and (b) lateral films post external fixation and pinning

distal radius to the metaphysis. Three 0.054 in. Kirschner wires (k-wires) were then placed from the radial styloid into the shaft of the radius. This allowed for adequate reduction of the fracture. To help maintain the reduction, a spanning external fixator was used across the wrist. This was secured with two 3 mm threaded pins in the index metacarpal and two 4 mm pins in the radial shaft along the dorsal-radial aspect of the forearm–wrist–hand. Fluoroscopy confirmed adequate reduction, hardware placement, and that the wrist was appropriately distracted. Passive finger flexion was easily achievable following fixation.

Clinical Course and Outcome

Following fixation, the pins sites were dressed with Xeroform and a bulky dressing with a sugar-tong splint was applied. Finger motion was allowed and encouraged right away following surgery. A below elbow splint was applied for 2 weeks post-surgery. Pin care was instructed to be performed daily. She was discouraged from any strenuous activity. The pins and external fixator were removed in the office at 6 weeks following surgery. While instructed to continue splinting, wrist motion was initiated at that time. As she regained wrist motion, strengthening and progression toward activity as tolerated was started at 10 weeks following surgery. At 1 year post surgery, the patient had wrist flexion and extension of 70 and 70 respectively, compared to 80 and 80 on the contralateral side. Radial and ulnar deviation was similar at 10° and 40° bilaterally. Her grip strength was 22 kg on right versus 24 on the left. Her DASH score was 11. Radiographs at 1 year are illustrated in Fig. 12.3a, b.

Literature Review and Discussion

Distal radius fractures are extremely common and represent the second most common fracture presenting to the emergency room. While quite common in osteoporotic and osteopenic populations,

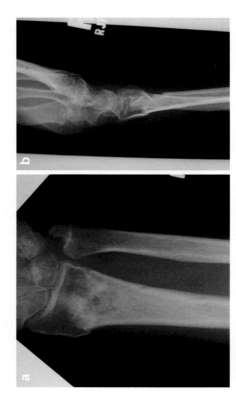

Fig. 12.3 (**a**) PA and (**b**) lateral films 1 year postop demonstrate healed fracture and adequate alignment. The patient was pain free with functional range of motion and returned to pre-injury activity levels

the injury affects all age groups. Many of these fractures can be treated nonoperatively with closed reduction and immobilization. Cases where closed reduction cannot be achieved or maintained are an indication for surgical reduction and stabilization. In addition, patients with higher functional demands likely benefit from a more anatomic reduction that may require surgical intervention. Varied surgical treatments and techniques have been described over the years. While the advent of locking plate technology, low profile dorsal plates and fragment specific fixation has reduced its use, external fixation and percutaneous pinning remains a valued treatment option and technique for these injuries.

The indications for external fixation and pinning include intra- and extra-articular dorsally angulated distal radius fractures that fail closed reduction. In addition, severely comminuted distal radius fractures, open fractures, and fracture/dislocations of the wrist would be considered indications for external fixation. Volarly angulated (e.g., Smith, volar Barton, and lunate facet type) fractures are more difficult to pin and maintain the reduction with an external fixator. Additional relative contraindications include patients with aversion to the presence of an external fixator or patients with poor compliance or lack of means to return for follow-up care.

Different types of external fixators are currently available. There are uniplanar and multiplanar devices. In addition, while most span the radiocarpal joint, others do not bridge the joint. The non-bridging devices have the advantage of allowing wrist motion while in place, but are generally reserved for extra-articular fractures and for patients with better bone quality. For cases with extensive comminution or osteoporotic bone, bridging external fixators are preferred.

Multiple factors will enhance or affect the strength and rigidity of the external fixation device. Pin size affects the strength. Pins with longer threads, conical design, and partial threads reduce the risk of failure. Pin placement also can influence the stability of the fixator. Insertion of more pins, placing pins close to the fracture, and larger spacing between pins will increase the rigidity of the construct. The alignment, size and position of the fixator bars will influence the fixator as well. Larger diameter bars, placing the bar of the fixator closer to the bone, stacking of bars, and placement of bars in multiple planes will strengthen the device.

Outcomes of external fixation have been favorable. Cooney et al. described the outcomes of 60 patients treated with external pin fixation and noted that 92 % of patients had no pain and 89 % had no deformity [1]. The authors concluded good or excellent results occurred in 90 % of cases.

Some studies have examined the use of external fixator with bone grafting. Leung et al. reviewed their outcomes of 100 cases of distal radius fractures treated with external fixation and iliac crest bone grafting with an average 20-month follow-up period [2]. The patients were treated uniformly and the devices were removed at 3 weeks. The average flexion and extension arc of motion was greater than 60° and 60°, respectively. In addition, maintenance of radiographic parameters was quite good. Cannegieter and Juttmann performed a prospective analysis of 32 cases of Colles' fractures treated with external fixator and cancellous bone grafting [3]. The fixators were left in place for 5 weeks. At a mean follow-up of 3 years, all patients had satisfactory functional outcomes, none had pain and all were satisfied with the result. However, five cases of radiographic malunion developed. Seven patients experienced complex regional pain syndrome.

A number of studies suggest that pinning in addition to external fixation yields better outcomes than external fixation alone. Fernandez and Geissler found that anatomic reduction could not be achieved or maintained with external fixation alone in a review of 40 cases and excellent radiographic and clinical outcomes were achieved with supplemental k-wire fixation [4]. Trumble et al. examined their outcomes of patients treated with Kapandji pinning alone versus those with supplemental external fixation [5]. The authors noted that elderly patients and those with volar and dorsal comminution had better outcomes when treated with supplemental external fixation. Lin et al. reviewed 20 cases of patients treated with external fixator alone versus 36 with external fixation and k-wires. Clinical and radiographic outcomes were superior in the group treated with external fixation and pinning [6].

There are several comparative studies between external fixation with other treatment methods over the last two decades. Many of the more recent analyses compare external fixation with fixed angle volar locking plates. Wright et al. reported their experience with treatment of distal radius fractures with fixed angle volar plating and external fixation [7]. At an average nearly 4-year follow-up period, the disability of the Arm, Shoulder, and Hand Questionnaire (DASH) scores were similar between the groups. While radiographic parameters were improved in the ORIF group, the two groups were comparable with respect to motion and strength was improved in the patients treated with external fixation. Rizzo et al. performed a similar comparison between locked volar plating in 41 patients to external fixation in 14 patients at a minimum of 2-year follow-up [8]. DASH, ulnar variance, and volar tilt were superior in the ORIF group. However, pain, grip strength, and range of motion (ROM) between groups at final evaluation were similar.

More recently there have been prospective studies examining outcomes between groups. Egol et al. prospectively randomized 88 patients to external fixation or locked volar plating [9]. Although the ORIF group showed early improvement of ROM, at 1 year this benefit diminished over time. In addition, there were no clinical, functional, or radiographic differences between the two groups. The authors concluded that there was no clear advantage of any treatment, but fewer reoperations were necessary in the external fixation group. Kreder et al. reported on a prospective review of outcomes between external fixation and ORIF, this multi-center study included 179 patients who were randomized between ORIF and external fixation groups [10]. Patients were followed for 2 years and the outcomes demonstrated similar improvements in pain and range of motion among groups. Interestingly, the external fixation group had superior functional outcome and earlier return to function. Finally, Rozental et al. prospectively analyzed outcomes between ORIF with locked volar plating and percutaneous pinning and external fixation or casting [11]. Twenty-two patients underwent closed reduction and pinning and 23 were treated with ORIF. DASH scores and motion were superior in the ORIF group at 6, 9, and 12 weeks post-surgery. However, at 1 year post-surgery, these results were similar between groups. They concluded that, while better results in the short term are expected in patients treated with ORIF using volar locking plates, both methods are effective for the treatment of dorsally angulated distal radius fractures.

Clinical Pearls/Pitfalls

Pearls

- Generally speaking, there are two methods of combing limited internal fixation with k-wires and external fixation: (1) initially facilitate reduction of the fracture fragments with k-wires +/− bone grafting and then apply fixator to span and maintain the reduction or (2) first span the fracture with the external fixator and then reduce and pin the fracture fragments +/− bone grafting. Our preference is (1).
- The more common pin placements include: (1) radial styloid pinning (usually with 0.054 or 0.062 in. k-wires), (2) Kapandji pins from dorsum of radius inserted through the fracture aiming proximally to buttress the reduction (0.054 or 0.062 in. wires), and (3) subchondral wires from the radial styloid (0.045 in. wires).
- Radial styloid pinning is best performed first and "fanning" or diverging the wires from styloid to engage the proximal radial diaphysis will help to strengthen the stability of the construct.
- A small incision over radial styloid allows for safe retraction of the superficial branch of the radial nerve while pinning.
- In addition, placing the wire driver in oscillate mode will minimize risk of capturing the nerve in the soft tissues as you drill.
- Use of fluoroscopy is helpful in confirming the reduction and pin placements.
- Since the subchondral pins are anchored at the radial styloid, they are best placed after securing and reducing the styloid.
- Kapandji pinning is usually best performed with two pins, one on either side of the 4th extensor compartment tendons.
- When securing the external fixator distally

  - A high speed, low torque drill for pre-drilling allows for better stability for pins
  - Make an incision over the dorsal-radial aspect of the index metacarpal and allow for visualization of branches of the superficial radial nerve.
  - Engaging the third metacarpal with the proximal pin will enhance the stability of the pin as the proximal index metacarpal will have weaker bone than the metacarpal shaft.

- When securing the fixator proximally

  - Incision approximately 8–10 cm from the radiocarpal joint can be made to expose the soft tissues and protect the tendons and radial nerve.
  - Place pins between ECRB and ECRL to avoid injury/irritation of superficial branch of the radial nerve, which exits from beneath the brachioradialis.
  - Pre-drilling can help avoid heat necrosis (especially in younger patients)—reduces risk of pin loosening.

- Close the external fixator pin wounds without tension.
- Close the skin incisions prior to placing the external fixator connecting bar/device to avoid difficulty in working around this during skin closure.
- Splinting the wrist, even in the presence of the fixator, with a thermoplastic splint allows for access to the pins (for pin care) and also supports the construct, minimizing micromotion of the pins.
- Use of dorsal bone grafting can provide structural support to the fracture and allow for maintenance of the reduction.

Pitfalls

- Avoid using an external fixator alone (without supplemental internal k-wire fixation) as it has been shown to have difficulty maintaining the reduction compared to external fixation and pinning [5, 12].
- Avoid overdistraction of the fixator. This can be avoided by ensuring that full passive finger motion is achievable. In addition, radiographs should demonstrate equidistant spaces between the radiocarpal and midcarpal joints.
- Avoid excessive flexion and ulnar deviation of the wrist. Adjustable fixators can help reposition the wrist following reduction.
- Pin site drainage can result in serious infections. This can be avoided by splinting, good pin care, and surveillance.

Conclusion

External fixation and percutaneous pinning, in its various forms, remains a valuable surgical treatment in the management of unstable distal radius fractures. Proper understanding of the principles of external fixation is critical in ensuring reliable outcomes and minimizing complications. While its indications continue to evolve, proper knowledge and comfort utilizing this technique will enhance the surgeon's ability to better manage this common injury.

References

1. Cooney 3rd WP, Linscheid RL, Dobyns JH. External pin fixation for unstable Colles' fractures. J Bone Joint Surg Am. 1979;61(6A):840–5.
2. Leung KS, Shen WY, Tsang HK, et al. An effective treatment of comminuted fractures of the distal radius. J Hand Surg [Am]. 1990;15(1):11–7.
3. Cannegieter DM, Juttmann JW. Cancellous grafting and external fixation for unstable Colles' fractures. J Bone Joint Surg Br. 1997;79(3):428–32.
4. Fernandez DL, Geissler WB. Treatment of displaced articular fractures of the radius. J Hand Surg [Am]. 1991;16(3):375–84.
5. Trumble TE, Wagner W, Hanel DP, et al. Intrafocal (Kapandji) pinning of distal radius fractures with and without external fixation. J Hand Surg [Am]. 1998;23(3):381–94.
6. Lin C, Sun JS, Hou SM. External fixation with or without supplementary intramedullary Kirschner wires in the treatment of distal radial fractures. Can J Surg. 2004;47(6):431–7.
7. Wright TW, Horodyski M, Smith DW. Functional outcome of unstable distal radius fractures: ORIF with a volar fixed-angle tine plate versus external fixation. J Hand Surg [Am]. 2005;30(2):289–99.
8. Rizzo M, Carothers JT, Kaat BA. Comparison of locked volar plating versus pinning and external fixation in the treatment of unstable intraarticular distal radius fractures. Hand. 2008;3(2):111–7.
9. Egol K, Walsh M, Tejwani N, et al. Bridging external fixation and supplementary Kirschner-wire fixation versus volar locked plating for unstable fractures of the distal radius: a randomised, prospective trial. J Bone Joint Surg. 2008;90(9):1214–21.
10. Kreder HJ, Hanel DP, Agel J, et al. Indirect reduction and percutaneous fixation versus open reduction and internal fixation for displaced intra-articular fractures of the distal radius: a randomised, controlled trial. J Bone Joint Surg Br. 2005;87(6):829–36.

11. Rozental TD, Blazar PE, Franko OI, et al. Functional outcomes for unstable distal radial fractures treated with open reduction and internal fixation or closed reduction and percutaneous fixation. A prospective randomized trial. J Bone Joint Surg Am. 2009;91(8):1837–46.
12. Sanders RA, Keppel FL, Waldrop JI. External fixation of distal radial fractures: results and complications. J Hand Surg [Am]. 1991;16(3):385–91.

Chapter 13
Ulnar Styloid Fracture with Distal Radioulnar Joint Instability

Nikhil R. Oak, Caroline N. Wolfe, and Jeffrey N. Lawton

Case Presentation

A 27-year-old, active, left-hand-dominant male fell from a truck bed onto an outstretched left arm. Initial radiographs revealed a distal radius fracture with an accompanying ulnar styloid fracture. Posteroanterior view demonstrated an impacted, comminuted distal radius fracture with articular extension as well as a concomitant fracture through the base of the ulnar styloid (Fig. 13.1). Ulnar styloid fracture demonstrated greater than 2 mm of radial displacement. Mild volar angulation was demonstrated on the lateral view (Fig. 13.2). The fracture was reduced and splinted in the emergency department.

The patient underwent open reduction and volar locking-plate fixation of his distal radius fracture. The distal radioulnar joint (DRUJ) during intraoperatively ballotment testing was found to be unstable. Open reduction and internal fixation of the ulnar styloid fracture was then performed using a tension-band technique. The DRUJ was then confirmed to be stable after repeat intraoperative testing (Fig. 13.3).

N.R. Oak, MD • C.N. Wolfe, MD (✉) • J.N. Lawton, MD
Department of Orthopaedic Surgery, University of Michigan Health System, A. Alfred Taubman Health Care Center, Floor 2, Reception: B, 2912 Taubman Center, 1500 East Medical Center Drive, Ann Arbor, MI 48109-5328, USA
e-mail: nikhiloak@gmail.com; wcarolin@med.umich.edu

© Springer International Publishing Switzerland 2016   165
J.N. Lawton (ed.), *Distal Radius Fractures*,
DOI 10.1007/978-3-319-27489-8_13

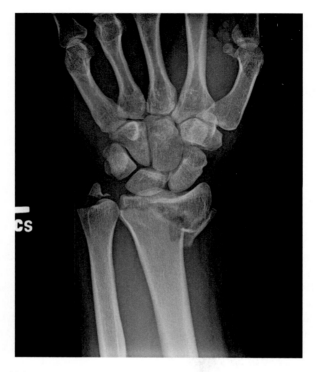

Fig. 13.1 Posteroanterior (PA) radiograph of left arm demonstrating an impacted, comminuted distal radius fracture with articular extension as well as a concomitant fracture through the base of the ulnar styloid with greater than 2 mm of radial displacement

Background

Ulnar styloid fractures accompany approximately 50–65 % of distal radius fractures. Their contribution to functional and clinical outcomes remains unclear. Several studies report that associated ulnar styloid fractures may not have an impact on anatomic, radiographic, or functional results [1–6]. In contrast, many studies have shown that these fractures are associated with DRUJ instability and triangular fibrocartilage complex (TFCC) tears [7–9].

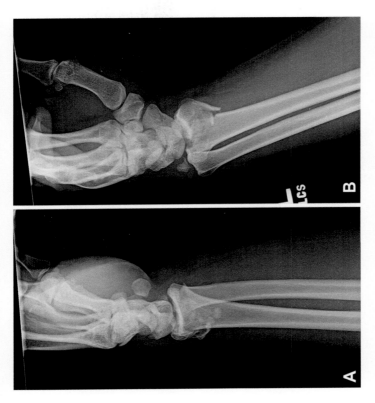

Fig. 13.2 (a) Lateral radiograph with mild volar angulation of the distal radius fracture. (b) Oblique lateral demonstrating ulnar styloid displacement of 3–4 mm as well as volar distal radial displacement and articular step-off

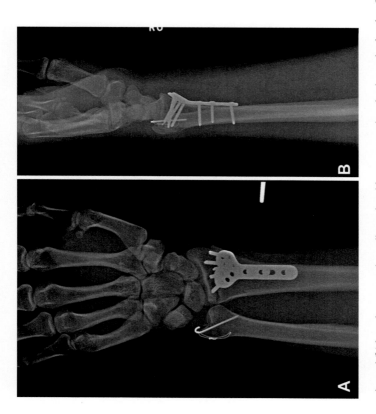

Fig. 13.3 (**a**) Posteroanterior and (**b**) lateral postoperative radiographs with near anatomic reduction and volar plate fixation of the distal radius fracture, and reduction and internal fixation of the ulnar styloid fracture using the tension-band technique

DRUJ instability affects approximately 3–37 % of distal radius fractures and can lead to long-term complications such as decreased forearm range of motion or strength, and chronic ulnar-sided wrist pain [7]. Proximity of the major DRUJ stabilizers to an ulnar styloid fracture raises concerns when a distal radius fracture is associated with an ulnar styloid fracture.

Anatomy

The ulna is the fixed element of the forearm. The DRUJ not only contributes to rotation of the radius about the ulna but also provides some axial and translational motion. For example, axial shortening and palmar translation of the radius relative to the ulna occur during forearm pronation [10, 11].

Stability of the DRUJ is well documented and is provided through bony anatomy as well as soft tissue stabilizers. The ulnar head is much smaller in circumference than the arc of the sigmoid notch, with the bony articulation contributing only 20 % of the stability [12]. Axial and translational motion changes the articular contact between the ulnar head and sigmoid notch, limiting the bony contribution to stability during extreme pronation or supination. Therefore, soft tissue constrains have a very important role in DRUJ stability [11].

The TFCC is the primary stabilizer of the DRUJ [7, 13–15]. Components of the TFCC include the triangular fibrocartilage proper (articular disc), the meniscus homologue (ulnocarpal meniscus), the ulnar collateral ligament, the dorsal and volar radioulnar ligament, and the sheath of the extensor carpi ulnaris (ECU) [14]. Secondary stabilizers include the interosseous membrane, the ECU and its subsheath, the joint capsule, and the pronator quadratus [7, 14]. Palmer and Werner [15] tested the contribution of the TFCC to DRUJ stability and found that sectioning of the TFCC led to dislocation of the joint in nearly all forearm positions, whereas sectioning of the pronator quadratus and capsule did not [15]. Within the TFCC, the dorsal and palmar radioulnar ligaments are responsible for a large portion of stability [11]. The radioulnar ligaments arise from the dorsal and palmar margin of the sigmoid notch and converge to insert onto the base of the ulnar styloid and the fovea. The superficial fibers of the radioulnar ligaments insert onto the base of the ulnar styloid and the deep fibers insert onto the fovea [7, 10, 14, 15]. In pronation, the superficial fibers of the dorsal ligament and the deep fibers of the palmar ligament become taut and constrain the joint. In supination the reverse occurs [7, 10, 11]. It is thought that disruption of the styloid may subsequently lead to laxity in the radioulnar ligaments of the TFCC leading to instability of the DRUJ.

DRUJ Instability

Ulnar styloid fractures are commonly associated with distal radius fractures but effects upon functional outcome and chronic instability of the DRUJ are unclear [16]. In addition, an associated TFCC tear with injury to the radioulnar ligaments can contribute to DRUJ instability following distal radius fractures in 7–33 % of cases [3, 17]. Stoffelen et al. [9] described that ulnar styloid fractures have a negative effect upon outcome because of their effect on the function of the DRUJ, reporting 13 of 272 patients had DRUJ instability after distal radius fractures. All 13 of these patients had a fracture of the ulnar styloid [9]. Oskarsson et al. [8] reported a case series of 158 distal radius fractures treated nonsurgically. They found that ulnar styloid involvement was a greater predictor of instability than articular involvement [8]. May et al. [7] described patterns and characteristics of ulnar styloid fracture, including size and displacement, to determine relative contribution to DRUJ instability when accompanying a distal radius fracture. During a 1-year interval, 166 distal radius fractures were retrospectively reviewed to determine potential negative impact on outcome. The authors reported that presence of an ulnar styloid fracture involving the base or with displacement more than 2 mm was a risk factor of DRUJ instability, not simply the presence of an ulnar styloid fracture itself [7].

In a prospective study of 138 patients with distal radius fractures treated with open reduction and rigid fixation using volar locking compression plates, Kim et al. [16] did not find a significant relationship between wrist functional outcomes and ulnar styloid fracture level or the amount of displacement. They concluded that an accompanying ulnar styloid fracture in patients with stable fixation of a distal radius fracture has no apparent adverse effect on wrist function or stability of the DRUJ. No differences may relate to indirect reduction of the ulnar styloid fracture after anatomic radius fixation. However, maintenance of an anatomic reduction of the distal radius fracture should be considered a prerequisite for non-operative treatment of ulnar styloid fractures [16].

Outcomes of Ulnar Styloid Nonunion

Approximately 25 % of ulnar styloid fractures fail to achieve bone union when left untreated [1, 7]. Again, the impact of nonunion on functional outcomes remains unclear. Tsukazaki and Iwasaki [18] reported nonunion in 13 of 17 patients with DRUJ instability. In 1996, Hauck and colleagues [19] classified nonunions based on the location of the styloid fracture. They recommended open reduction and internal fixation of ulnar styloid fractures in type 2 fracture nonunions, where the fracture includes radioulnar insertion site [19].

On the contrary, several studies show ulnar styloid nonunion does not affect wrist functional outcomes, ulnar-sided wrist pain, or DRUJ stability when the distal radius fracture is fixed [1, 2, 20]. In a prospective cohort of 144 patients, Sammer et al. [1] examined the outcome of untreated ulnar styloid fractures after volar plating of distal radius fractures and DRUJ stability was confirmed. Sixty-one percent of the cohort had a styloid fracture. Patients with a stable DRUJ after fixation of the distal radius maintained stability. A nonunion rate of 68 % was reported but the presence, size, displacement, or healing status of the ulnar styloid fracture did not affect functional scores or DRUJ stability [1].

Buijze and Ring [2] reported a 56 % nonunion rate in 36 patients with fractures of both the distal radius and proximal half of the ulnar styloid who underwent volar plate fixation of the distal radius and no repair of the styloid fracture. They found that nonunion of the ulnar styloid had no effect on wrist function, pain, or upper extremity-specific health status [2]. Kim et al. [20] evaluated the functional and radiographic outcomes of 91 patients with a distal radius fracture and accompanying ulnar styloid fracture who underwent volar locking-plate fixation of the distal radius. They reported union in 21 % of patients but no difference in functional outcomes, ulnar-sided wrist pain, or DRUJ stability [20].

Surgical Technique

Various methods of ulnar styloid fixation have been described, including Kirschner wires, tension-band wiring, compression screws, variable-pitch headless screws, mini-fragment plates, and suture anchors. The presented case was fixed using tension-band technique. The ulnar styloid is typically approached just palmar and parallel to the ECU tendon. One or two oblique Kirschner wires are inserted through the styloid tip. A 24-gauge-tension band is passed around the tip of the wire and, in a figure-of-eight fashion, through a hole in the ulnar neck [21].

Conclusion

A distal radius fracture with associated ulnar styloid fracture may place the patient at higher risk for DRUJ instability. With anatomic reduction and volar plate fixation of the distal radius fracture, the ulnar styloid fracture is often indirectly reduced and the DRUJ remains stable. It has been shown that ulnar styloid fracture or its nonunion does not affect outcome with adequate reduction and fixation of the distal radius fracture. However, large ulnar styloid base fractures or displacement over 2 mm may require open reduction and fixation of the ulnar styloid fracture to achieve DRUJ stability due to the proximity of major DRUJ stabilizing ligaments. DRUJ instability may lead to chronic pain, decreased range of motion, and need for further salvage procedures for relief. The most important guiding principle is to evaluate DRUJ stability following distal radius fixation routinely to determine whether or not to address concomitant ulnar styloid fracture. If the DRUJ remains stable after anatomic fixation of the distal radius, ulnar styloid fixation is rarely required. If the DRUJ remains unstable, we would recommend open reduction and internal fixation of ulnar styloid fracture to achieve stability and reduce the risk of long-term problems.

References

1. Sammer DM, Shah HM, Shauver MJ, Chung KC. The effect of ulnar styloid fractures on patient-rated outcomes after volar locking plating of distal radius fractures. J Hand Surg Am. 2009;34(9):1595–602.
2. Buijze GA, Ring D. Clinical impact of United versus nonunited fractures of the proximal half of the ulnar styloid following volar plate fixation of the distal radius. J Hand Surg Am. 2010;35(2):223–7.
3. Lindau T, Adlercreutz C, Aspenberg P. Peripheral tears of the triangular fibrocartilage complex cause distal radioulnar joint instability after distal radial fractures. J Hand Surg Am. 2000;25(3):464–8.
4. Lindau T, Hagberg L, Adlercreutz C, Jonsson K, Aspenberg P. Distal radioulnar instability is an independent worsening factor in distal radial fractures. Clin Orthop Relat Res. 2000;376:229–35.
5. af Ekenstam F, Jakobsson OP, Wadin K. Repair of the triangular ligament in Colles' fracture. No effect in a prospective randomized study. Acta Orthop Scand. 1989;60(4):393–6.
6. Souer JS, Ring D, Matschke S, Audige L, Marent-Huber M, Jupiter JB. Effect of an unrepaired fracture of the ulnar styloid base on outcome after plate-and-screw fixation of a distal radial fracture. J Bone Joint Surg Am. 2009;91(4):830–8.
7. May MM, Lawton JN, Blazar PE. Ulnar styloid fractures associated with distal radius fractures: incidence and implications for distal radioulnar joint instability. J Hand Surg Am. 2002;27(6):965–71.
8. Oskarsson GV, Aaser P, Hjall A. Do we underestimate the predictive value of the ulnar styloid affection in Colles fractures? Arch Orthop Trauma Surg. 1997;116(6–7):341–4.

9. Stoffelen D, De Smet L, Broos P. The importance of the distal radioulnar joint in distal radial fractures. J Hand Surg Br. 1998;23(4):507–11.

10. Sammer DM, Chung KC. Management of the distal radioulnar joint and ulnar styloid fracture. Hand Clin. 2012;28(2):199–206.

11. Ward LD, Ambrose CG, Masson MV, Levaro F. The role of the distal radioulnar ligaments, interosseous membrane, and joint capsule in distal radioulnar joint stability. J Hand Surg Am. 2000;25(2):341–51.

12. Huang JI, Hanel DP. Anatomy and biomechanics of the distal radioulnar joint. Hand Clin. 2012;28(2):157–63.

13. Shaw JA, Bruno A, Paul EM. Ulnar styloid fixation in the treatment of posttraumatic instability of the radioulnar joint: a biomechanical study with clinical correlation. J Hand Surg Am. 1990;15(5):712–20.

14. Palmer AK, Werner FW. The triangular fibrocartilage complex of the wrist–anatomy and function. J Hand Surg Am. 1981;6(2):153–62.

15. Palmer AK, Werner FW. Biomechanics of the distal radioulnar joint. Clin Orthop Relat Res. 1984;187:26–35.

16. Kim JK, Koh YD, Do NH. Should an ulnar styloid fracture be fixed following volar plate fixation of a distal radial fracture? J Bone Joint Surg Am. 2010;92(1):1–6.

17. Fujitani R, Omokawa S, Akahane M, Iida A, Ono H, Tanaka Y. Predictors of distal radioulnar joint instability in distal radius fractures. J Hand Surg Am. 2011;36(12):1919–25.

18. Tsukazaki T, Iwasaki K. Ulnar wrist pain after Colles' fracture. 109 fractures followed for 4 years. Acta Orthop Scand. 1993;64(4):462–4.

19. Hauck RM, Skahen 3rd J, Palmer AK. Classification and treatment of ulnar styloid nonunion. J Hand Surg Am. 1996;21(3):418–22.

20. Kim JK, Yun YH, Kim DJ, Yun GU. Comparison of united and nonunited fractures of the ulnar styloid following volar-plate fixation of distal radius fractures. Injury. 2011;42(4):371–5.

21. Adams BD. Distal radioulnar joint instability. In: Wolfe SW, editor. Green's operative hand surgery. 6th ed. Philadelphia: Saunders/Elsevier; 2011. p. 523–60.

Chapter 14
Distal Radius Fractures with Ulnar Head and Neck Fractures

Kristofer S. Matullo and David G. Dennison

Case Presentation

AC is a 52-year-old right-hand dominant homemaker who was involved in a motor vehicle accident as a restrained passenger. She complained of pain to the right distal forearm without loss of sensation. On examination, there was a 3 cm wound overlying the ulnar border of the right distal forearm with exposed bone but viable surrounding soft tissues and she had an intact neurovascular examination. Radiographs (Fig. 14.1a, b) demonstrate a comminuted, extra-articular metadiaphyseal fracture of the distal radius (AO type A3) and an open Gustilo Anderson grade II ulnar neck fracture (type Q2) [1, 2]. The patient underwent urgent surgical intervention with no other injuries and well controlled hypertension.

K.S. Matullo, MD (✉)
Department of Orthopaedic Surgery, St. Luke's University Health
Network, Bethlehem, PA 18015, USA
e-mail: Kristofer.Matullo@sluhn.org

D.G. Dennison, MD
Department of Orthopedic Surgery, Mayo Clinic, Rochester,
MN 55905, USA

© Springer International Publishing Switzerland 2016   175
J.N. Lawton (ed.), *Distal Radius Fractures*,
DOI 10.1007/978-3-319-27489-8_14

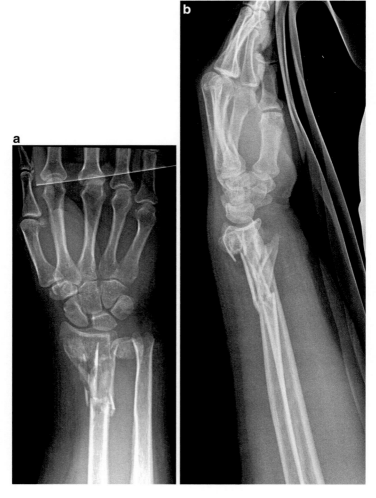

Fig. 14.1 PA (**a**) and lateral (**b**) radiograph demonstrate a comminuted, extra-articular metadiaphyseal fracture of the distal radius with a concomitant ulnar neck fracture

Literature Review

Fractures of the distal radius with concomitant ulnar neck or head fractures occur in approximately 6 % of patients. Forty-six percent of these patients having abnormalities of the distal radioulnar joint (DRUJ) [3]. Anatomic reduction of these fractures with restoration of the DRUJ is imperative to help restore stability and motion through the DRUJ, while trying to minimize the risk of posttraumatic osteoarthritis. A malunited fracture with the ulnar head located volar to the distal radioulnar joint leads to decreased pronation while a dorsally malunited ulnar head will lead to decreased supination compared to normal alignment [4]. Up to 16 % of patients may develop a synostosis between the radius and ulna in these fracture patterns [3].

Classification of ulnar head and neck fractures uses a Q modifier within the Comprehensive Classification of Fractures. Type Q1 fractures involve the base of the ulnar styloid; ulnar neck fractures are type Q2 without comminution or Q3 with comminution; Q4 are ulnar head fractures; combination ulnar head and neck fractures are Q5, and more proximal shaft fractures are type Q6 [2].

Fractures of the distal radius with ulnar head or shaft may be stabilized by a variety of methods. Fixation of the distal radius utilizes standard techniques, such as external fixation or open reduction and internal fixation (ORIF), while fixation of the distal ulna can be accomplished by a variety of methods. Kirschner wire (K-wire) fixation of the ulnar fragment to the shaft secures the fracture, but may be associated with pin site irritation or increased risk of infection (Fig. 14.2a, b). K-wire fixation is also limited by bone quality and has the best chance of maintaining fracture reduction in patients with fracture patterns that have minimal to no comminution [5].

The outcome of plate fixation was reported by Ring et al. in 2004 using a subcutaneous condylar plate along the ulnar border for stabilization of the ulnar fracture [2]. While this method produced good to excellent results in 21 of 24 patients, seven patients required removal of the ulnar plate due to irritation. Functional range of motion of the wrist was recovered with an average of 50° flexion, 52° extension, 76° supination, and 64° pronation, with no incidence of DRUJ instability.

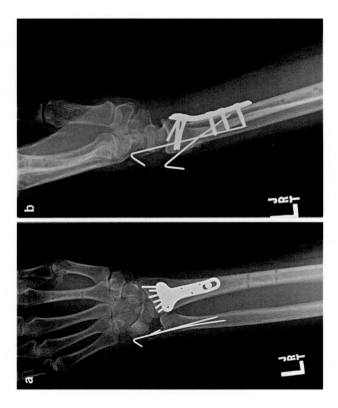

Fig. 14.2 PA (**a**) and lateral (**b**) radiograph demonstrating fixation of a distal radius fracture and ulnar styloid and neck fracture utilizing a locking, volar, distal radius plate and crossed K-wires

One other small series reported upon plate fixation utilizing locked, lower profile plates. All patients healed with a functional range of motion similar to Ring et al. [2], while two patients sustained a transient ulnar sensory neuropraxia which both resolved completely and no patients required hardware removal [5]. Comminuted ulnar fractures may be treated with dual plating utilizing a two-column method as described by Bessho et al. [6].

Specific plating systems for the distal ulna have been developed and evaluated. In a series of 25 patients with an average follow-up of 15 months, Lee et al. treated concomitant fractures of the distal radius and ulnar head/neck with a volar distal radius plate and a distal ulnar hook plate. The range of motion at final follow-up was 72° flexion, 69° extension, 77° pronation, 82° supination, 24° radial deviation, and 35° ulnar deviation. Grip strength measured between 80 and 91 % of the contralateral side. There were no wrists with DRUJ instability; however, four patients needed secondary bone graft placement for delayed union. Average DASH scores were reported at 14 with a modified Mayo wrist score of 87 [7]. Geissler reported his technique with a volarly placed distal ulnar plate to decrease irritation at the subcutaneous ulnar border in noncomminuted fractures with good results [8]. The plate must be placed proximally to the distal radioulnar joint with the screws projecting distally into the ulnar head fragment to avoid impingement at the sigmoid notch during supination and pronation, as the articular cartilage of the distal ulna covers a 270° arc [2, 8]. When considering the volar placement of the plate, the length of the screws should be measured carefully to avoid leaving the screw tip in the ECU groove, which may irritate the ECU tendon.

A direct comparison of patients with distal radius and distal ulnar fractures treated with ORIF of the distal radius and either ORIF versus closed reduction with or without pinning of the distal ulna was performed by Gschwentner et al. In this series, patients had improved flexion–extension arcs of 114° and pronation–supination arcs of 162° in the closed reduction group versus 77° and 107° in the ORIF group, respectively. There was no significant difference in grip strength or pain [9]. Methods to combine the lower profile pins and the stability of plating involve the usage of an intrafocal pin plate in the ulnar head or within subcapital fractures of the ulna [10].

Fractures with extensive levels of comminution may not be amenable to ORIF given the size or number of fracture fragments. In these cases, arthroplasty or resection may be necessary. While the data for arthroplasty is present [11], the literature demonstrates support for primary ulnar head resection [12–15]. In a case series of 15 patients followed for an average of 5.8 years, fractures of the distal radius and ulna were treated with external fixation with or without ORIF of the distal radius and simultaneous excision of the ulnar head. A "watertight" repair of the periosteal sleeve and TFCC complex provided stability to the DRUJ and ulnar carpus. Compared to the uninjured side, range of motion was equal or greater than 85 %, grip strength was 88.6 %, and there were no cases of DRUJ instability or ulnocarpal subluxation [14].

Treatment of the distal ulnar fracture with excision and a simultaneous extensor carpi ulnaris tenodesis through a dorsal ulnar incision was described in 11 patients with an average age of 62 and an average follow-up of 42 months. There were no cases of instability and results were graded as excellent in seven patients and good in four patients. Grip strength averaged 90 % of the contralateral side with range of motion of 105° in the flexion–extension arc and 158° in the pronation–supination arc. Immediate resection in elderly patients greater than 70 years of age yielded similar results with slightly reduced grip strength of 69 % compared to the contralateral side [15].

The level of the distal radius and ulna fracture may also predict instability at the DRUJ. The distal interosseous ligament and the variable presence of the distal oblique bundle also influence stability. Orbay has proposed a classification of instability based upon these anatomical factors and the observation that fractures of the radius and ulna can occur proximal, distal, or in variable levels relative to these structures [16]. While we may not know what soft tissue anatomy the patient has or exactly what is injured, we can reduce the fractures accurately and stabilize the DRUJ. In the operating room, the radius should be reduced anatomically. This includes correcting the coronal plane deformity to appropriately tension all soft tissue attachments. The ulna is also reduced and stabilized. If instability of the DRUJ persists, then TFC repair or ulnar styloid repair is necessary. Alternatively, the radius and ulna may be stabilized with cross pinning or a radioulnar external fixator in supination for 4–6 weeks [17].

Decision Making

The patient was brought urgently to the operating room, where an irrigation and debridement of the fracture was performed. The wound was clean and there was sufficient skin for primary closure so the surgical plan was to proceed with primary open reduction and internal fixation. The distal radius was approached through a trans-FCR approach and was reduced and then stabilized with a volar locking plate placed as a "bridging plate" to span the metadiaphyseal comminution.

After establishing the correct length and alignment by fixing the radius, the distal ulna was addressed. The traumatic laceration was extended proximally and distally along the subcutaneous ulnar border. The dorsal cutaneous branch of the ulnar nerve was identified and protected. The interval between the flexor carpi ulnaris (FCU) and ECU was developed. The ulnar head was reduced and stabilized with an ulnar hook plate with a simultaneous retrograde bicortical screw placed through the ulnar styloid. Interfragmentary compression was obtained and the plate was secured with nonlocking screws in the proximal ulnar shaft. The DRUJ was stable when tested in neutral, pronation, and supination.

The implants were chosen given the size of the fracture fragments and the bone quality. As the distal fragment was one piece, secure distal fixation could be achieved and therefore the fracture did not require primary arthroplasty or resection. Given the presence of the open wound, the traumatic soft tissue injury, as well as the size of the fragment, percutaneous pins potentially increase the risk of post-operative complications, such as perioperative infection. While the distal fracture fragment was large enough to allow for primary fracture fragment fixation, it was also too small for multiple screws to be placed within the ulnar head fragment. Therefore, the distal ulnar hook plate was selected and fixation was supplemented with a retrograde bicortical screw placed through the plate at the ulnar styloid.

Postoperatively, the patient was placed within a sugar-tong long arm splint for 2 weeks. At the first post-operative visit, the sutures were removed. The patient was placed into a removable Munster splint and received occupational therapy for active and active

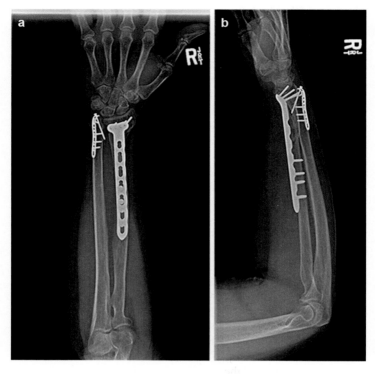

Fig. 14.3 PA (**a**) and lateral (**b**) radiograph demonstrate a well-healed distal radius and ulna fracture

assisted range of motion. At 6 weeks, the splint was discontinued and the patient was allowed more aggressive range of motion with progression to strengthening. Final evaluation 5 months after injury demonstrated a well-healed distal radius and ulna fracture (Fig. 14.3a, b), a stable distal radioulnar joint, and full composite fist formation. Final pronation/supination was 50/50° compared to 60/60° of the contralateral wrist with flexion of 50°, extension of 40°, radial deviation of 20°, and ulnar deviation of 38°.

Tips and Tricks

Establishing the length and alignment of the radius and ulna is paramount for adequate function postoperatively. We generally prefer to complete an anatomic reduction of the radius and the sigmoid notch first. The reduction of the volar-ulnar radius helps correct the length of the radius, the coronal plane alignment, and at least a portion of the sigmoid notch. Following reduction and fixation of the radius, the elbow can be flexed to 90° while maintaining the forearm in neutral rotation. This position can be maintained by use of finger-trap traction in a wrist arthroscopy tower which can allow simultaneous use of fluoroscopy as well. This will allow exposure of the ulnar head and neck through a medial subcutaneous approach between the FCU and ECU tendons. During the surgical dissection, identify and protect the dorsal cutaneous branch of the ulnar nerve, as injury to this structure could result in postoperative numbness or a painful neuroma.

Exposure through the FCU/ECU interval allows fixation of the styloid, head, or neck of the ulna and can be extended for fixation of fractures that extend more proximally. This incision allows placement of the plate in a volar position if desired, as described by Geissler [8]. If the decision is made to resect the ulnar head or perform a primary arthroplasty, the distal incision may be curved dorsally if required. If the articular surface requires reduction, a dorsal exposure can be made through the floor of the fifth extensor tendon compartment. The proximal capsule is incised between the radius and ulna preserving the dorsal radioulnar ligament. The distal capsular incision continues 90° in the ulnar direction and just proximal to the dorsal radioulnar ligament and stops before the ECU tendon. This will allow wide exposure to the ulnar head, TFC, and sigmoid notch.

Kirschner wires may also be used for fixation to aid in both the reduction and stabilization of the individual fragments. After exposure, a K-wire may be inserted distal to the ulnar styloid to identify the most distal plate position. Also, utilization of a K-wire in the distal ulnar fragment as a joystick can assist with reduction and restoration of the correct rotation of the ulnar head. As a reference, the ulnar styloid and the olecranon should be palpable roughly within the same plane. After proper reduction and alignment are obtained, the K-wire may be advanced into the proximal ulna or the distal radius to stabilize the ulnar head fragment in its reduced position. If instability is noted with the proximal ulnar shaft fracture fragment, a temporary K-wire maybe driven from ulnar shaft into the radial shaft to help stabilize the fragment from excessive volar and dorsal translation, allowing for easier reduction of the distal ulnar head to the stabilized ulnar shaft. Cross pinning the radius and ulna can be helpful intra-operatively to obtain a reduction, but we prefer to then attempt to provide stable fixation and remove the cross pins if possible. If plate fixation of the ulnar head is to be utilized, remember that these are to be unicortical screws. A plate/screw construct that allows these screws to be locking is advantageous.

Digital range of motion and edema control are begun immediately in the post-operative period. When the ulna and DRUJ are rigidly stabilized, flexion, extension, pronation, and supination of the wrist may begin at about 10–14 days or at the first post-operative visit after evaluation of the radiograph and surgical wounds. With rigid fixation of the radius, if there is concern for stability of the DRUJ or the distal ulna, 3–4 weeks in a neutral forearm cast is usually sufficient to provide comfort and allow early healing of the distal ulna and radius. Following initial splint or cast immobilization a splint is typically provided for patient comfort until range of motion normalizes. Once the patient achieves pain-free rotation of 45° of pronation and 45° of supination, the splint is discontinued. Strengthening may progress as the patient becomes more comfortable within a functional range of motion.

References

1. Gustilo RB, Anderson JT. Prevention of infection in the treatment of one thousand and twenty-five open fractures of long bones: retrospective and prospective analyses. J Bone Joint Surg Am. 1976;58(4):453–8.
2. Ring D, McCarty LP, Campbell D, Jupiter JB. Condylar blade plate fixation of unstable fractures of the distal ulna associated with fracture of the distal radius. J Hand Surg Am. 2004;29(1):103–9.
3. Biyani A, Simison AJ, Klenerman L. Fractures of the distal radius and ulna. J Hand Surg Br. 1995;20(3):357–64.

4. Ishikawa J, Iwasaki N, Minami A. Influence of distal radioulnar joint subluxation on restricted forearm rotation after distal radius fracture. J Hand Surg Am. 2005;30(6):1178–84.

5. Dennison DG. Open reduction and internal locked fixation of unstable distal ulna fractures with concomitant distal radius fracture. J Hand Surg Am. 2007;32(6):801–5.

6. Bessho Y, Okazaki M, Nakamura T. Double plate fixation for correction of the malunited distal ulna fracture: a case report. Hand Surg. 2011;16(3): 335–7.

7. Lee SK, Kim KJ, Park JS, Choy WS. Distal ulna hook plate fixation for unstable distal ulna fracture associated with distal radius fracture. Orthopedics. 2012;35(9):e1358–64.

8. Geissler WB. Management distal radius and distal ulnar fractures with fragment specific plate. J Wrist Surg. 2013;2(2):190–4.

9. Gschwentner M, Arora R, Wambacher M, Gabl M, Lutz M. Distal forearm fracture in the adult: is ORIF of the radius and closed reduction of the ulna a treatment option in distal forearm fracture? Arch Orthop Trauma Surg. 2008;128(8):847–55.

10. Nemeth N, Bindra RR. Fixation of distal ulna fractures associated with distal radius fractures using intrafocal pin plate. J Wrist Surg. 2014;3(1): 55–9.

11. Grechenig W, Peicha G, Fellinger M. Primary ulnar head prosthesis for the treatment of an irreparable ulnar head fracture dislocation. J Hand Surg Br. 2001;26(3):269–71.

12. Pansard E, Chantelot C, Mares O. Fracture of the distal radius associated with an articular comminutive fracture of the distal ulna: treatment in emergency by osteosynthesis of the radius by volar locking plate for the radius and a resection of the distal end of the ulna: report of one case. Chir Main. 2011;30(1):69–72.

13. Ruchelsman DE, Raskin KB, Rettig ME. Outcome following acute primary distal ulna resection for comminuted distal ulna fractures at the time of operative fixation of unstable fractures of the distal radius. Hand (N Y). 2009;4(4):391–6.

14. Seitz Jr WH, Raikin SM. Resection of comminuted ulna head fragments with soft tissue reconstruction when associated with distal radius fractures. Tech Hand Up Extrem Surg. 2007;11(4):224–30.

15. Yoneda H, Watanabe K. Primary excision of the ulnar head for fractures of the distal ulna associated with fractures of the distal radius in severe osteoporotic patients. J Hand Surg Eur Vol. 2014;39(3):293–9.

16. Trehan SK, Orbay JL, Wolfe SW. Coronal shift of distal radius fractures: influence of the distal interosseous membrane on distal radioulnar joint instability. J Hand Surg Am. 2015;40(1):159–62.

17. Ruch DS, Lumsden BC, Papadonikolakis A. Distal radius fractures: a comparison of tension band wiring versus ulnar outrigger external fixation for the management of distal radioulnar instability. J Hand Surg Am. 2005;30(5):969–77.

Chapter 15
DRUJ Dislocation/Galeazzi Fracture

Caroline N. Wolfe and Jeffrey N. Lawton

Case Presentation

A 57-year-old right-hand-dominant woman presented after a fall in which she sustained an isolated, closed left forearm injury. Initial imaging demonstrated a >100 % displaced, radial shaft fracture with shortening and disruption of the distal radioulnar joint (DRUJ) (Fig. 15.1). The fracture was greater than 7.5 cm proximal from the midarticular surface of the radius. She underwent open reduction and internal fixation of radial shaft fracture. After fixation, the DRUJ was evaluated and confirmed to be stable. Postoperative radiographs demonstrated restoration of radial length and DRUJ congruity (Fig. 15.2). With a supervised therapy program, she regained full elbow/wrist and forearm range of motion and returned to full function (Fig. 15.3).

C.N. Wolfe (✉) J.N. Lawton, MD
Department of Orthopaedic Surgery, University of Michigan Health
System, A. Alfred Taubman Health Care Center, Floor 2, Reception: B,
2912 Taubman Center, 1500 East Medical Center Drive,
Ann Arbor, MI 48109-5328, USA
e-mail: wcarolin@med.umich.edu

© Springer International Publishing Switzerland 2016   187
J.N. Lawton (ed.), *Distal Radius Fractures*,
DOI 10.1007/978-3-319-27489-8_15

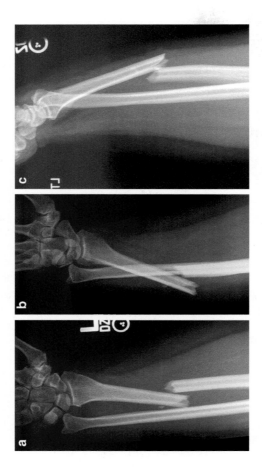

Fig. 15.1 (**a** and **b**) Radiographs demonstrating a left radial shaft fracture with 100 % displacement, radial shortening, and disruption of the distal radioulnar joint (DRUJ). The fracture appears to be greater than 7.5 cm from midarticular surface of the radius. (**c**) On lateral X-ray, the radius appeared shortened and displaced volar, creating disruption of the DRUJ

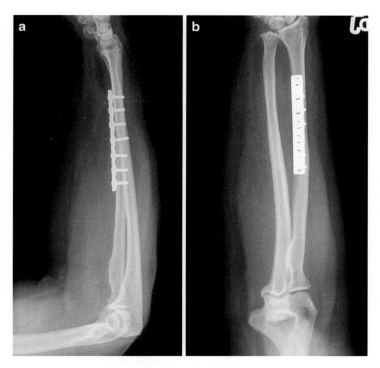

Fig. 15.2 The patient underwent stable fixation of the radial shaft fracture with compression plating. After fixation, the distal radioulnar joint (DRUJ) was tested and appeared stable. Postoperative radiographs (**a** and **b**) demonstrate restoration of radial length and DRUJ congruity

Background

A fracture of the shaft of the radius concomitant with a dislocation of the DRUJ is referred to as a Galeazzi fracture-dislocation. It is a fairly uncommon injury, making up 3 % to 7 % of all forearm fractures [1]. This fracture-dislocation is very unstable and the disruption of the DRUJ is often unappreciated during initial evaluation [2]. Persistent instability of the DRUJ leads to pain at the wrist and restricted forearm rotation [3]. Mistakes in treatment

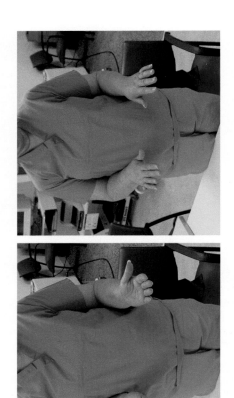

Fig. 15.3 The patient regained full forearm supination and pronation with decreased pain postoperatively

typically account for unsatisfactory results. Sir Astley Cooper was the first to describe this fracture-dislocation and the difficulty of reducing and maintaining reduction [4]. However, it was named after Italian surgeon Riccardo Galeazzi of Milan, Italy [5]. In 1934 he presented a series of 18 patients and elaborated on the incidence, pathomechanics, and management. He managed these fractures by closed reduction and splinting but his results were suboptimal with recurrence in DRUJ disruption [5]. He was the first to appreciate that the radius fracture was linked to the DRUJ disruption and that both needed to be addressed [6–10].

Anatomy and Biomechanics

The DRUJ is a complex articulation between the ulnar head and sigmoid notch of the distal radius, contributing to forearm pronation and supination. Stability is provided through a combination of bony architecture and soft tissue constraints. The ulnar head is much smaller in circumference than the arc of the sigmoid notch, therefore, the bony articulation contributes to only 20 % of the stability [11]. The soft tissue structures are responsible for maintaining stability through forearm rotation, consisting of static constraints and dynamic muscle stabilizers. These stabilizers include the ligaments found in the triangular fibrocartilage complex (TFCC), the pronator quadratus, and the interosseous membrane (IOM) [12, 13].

It has been demonstrated that the TFCC is the primary stabilizer of the DRUJ. In 1984, Palmer and Werner [14] tested the contribution of the TFCC to DRUJ stability. They found that sectioning of the TFCC led to dislocation of the joint in nearly all forearm positions, whereas sectioning of the pronator quadratus and capsule did not [14]. Within the TFCC, the dorsal and palmar radioulnar ligaments are responsible for a large portion of stability. The radioulnar ligaments attach to the fovea and the ulnar styloid as the deep and superficial limbs, respectively [6], susceptible to injury with basilar styloid fractures. The dorsal radioulnar ligaments are tight in pronation while the palmar ligaments are tight in supination [6].

The IOM has been demonstrated to be a secondary stabilizer of the DRUJ. It is a complex ligamentous structure that transfers load from radius to ulna. The central band, the strongest portion of the IOM, plays an important role in stabilization of the forearm [6]. Furthermore, the IOM is essential to maintain DRUJ kinematics when the radioulnar ligaments and TFCC are sacrificed [15].

Classification

Various systems have been used to classify this injury. The mechanism of injury usually involves a high-velocity direct impact with axial loading of an outstretched arm.

The ulna is the fixed element of the forearm with the radius rotating about the ulna. In Galeazzi fractures, the ulna also remains fixed and the radius displaces relative to it. Unfortunately, however, depending on the age of literature, it can be described as either displacement of the radius or the ulna, which can be quite confusing.

In 1975, Dameron [16] subdivided these fractures into ulnar volar or ulnar dorsal. In 1987, observation by Walsh and colleagues [17] led to classification based on the displacement of the distal radius fragment and proposed mechanism of injury. They classified fracture-dislocations into type I and type II after observing dorsal displacement in 20 and volar displacement in 21 pediatric patients. Type I fractures, apex volar, result from axial loading of the forearm in supination and dorsal displacement of the distal radius. In type II fractures, apex dorsal, hyperpronation with axial loading causes the distal radius to displace volar [6, 17].

In 1994, Macule Beneyto and colleagues [2] classified the fracture-dislocation based on the distance of the radial fracture from the radial styloid. Type I injuries refer to fractures between 0 and 10 cm from the styloid process. Type two fractures occur between 10 and 15 cm, and type three fractures are more than 15 cm from the styloid process [2]. In their series of 33 patients with Galeazzi fractures, type I injuries were associated with worse results [2].

In 2001, Rettig and Raskin [9] introduced a clinically predictive classification system based on the probability of DRUJ instability after fracture fixation. In their retrospective review, the fracture was fixed and then the DRUJ was tested to determine if the distance of the fracture from the midarticular surface of the distal radius contributed to DRUJ instability and the need for further fixation. Galeazzi fractures were divided into type I or type II based on the distance of the fracture from the distal radius midarticular surface. Type I fractures were located in the distal third of the radius, within 7.5 cm of the midarticular surface of the distal radius. Type II fractures were within the middle third of the radial shaft, more than 7.5 cm from the midarticular surface of the distal radius [9]. The authors found that 55 % of type I fractures required DRUJ stabilization compared to 6 % of type II fractures [3, 9]. Therefore, according to Rettig and Raskin [9], fractures within 7.5 cm of the midarticular surface of the distal radius are more likely to require DRUJ stabilization.

Evaluation

Obvious deformity with angulation and shortening of the radial forearm and prominence of the ulnar head is usually appreciated on initial presentation. Patients may report local tenderness, swelling, and limited forearm motion. Any fracture to the distal third of radius should be regarded as potential Galeazzi fracture-dislocation with disruption of the DRUJ.

Initial radiographs should include posterior–anterior (PA) and lateral views of the wrist and elbow. In the PA view, widening or partial overlap of the radius and ulna can demonstrate dorsal or volar DRUJ dislocation [18]. The lateral view of the wrist is very important when considering DRUJ disruption, demonstrating subluxation of the ulnar head. It is important to analyze a true lateral wrist X-ray when determining disruption. On a true lateral view of the wrist, the pisiform overlaps the distal pole of the scaphoid [19]. On a poor lateral view of the wrist, as seen in Fig. 15.4a, the DRUJ appears to be disrupted. However, when looking closely, the pisiform and the distal pole of the scaphoid do not overlap. Looking at the same patient in Fig. 15.4b, a true lateral displays overlap of the pisiform and the distal pole of the scaphoid and the DRUJ is confirmed to be reduced.

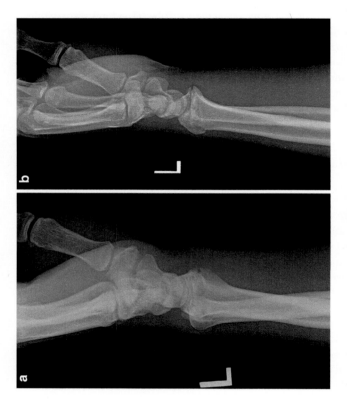

Fig. 15.4 (a) False lateral in which the distal radioulnar joint (DRUJ) appears "disrupted"—Note no overlap of the pisiform and distal pole of the scaphoid. (b) True lateral—Note overlap of the pisiform and distal pole of the scaphoid. DRUJ is reduced. This is the same patient shown in Fig. 15.1a

The amount of radial shortening on X-rays may also help predict the amount of soft tissue injury. Schneiderman and colleagues [20] presented a cadaveric study in which an osteotomy of the radius was performed, followed by different orders of soft tissue transection to determine the correlation of the amount of shortening of the radius to the amount of soft tissue injury. When performing a radial osteotomy alone, they found approximately 5 mm of shortening. Five to 10 mm of shortening was observed after transection of the TFCC or IOM in combination with a radial osteotomy. Shortening greater than 10 mm required a radial osteotomy with transection of both the TFCC and IOM. Therefore, radial shortening greater than 5 mm should increase suspicion of injury to either the TFCC or IOM [20]. Contralateral X-rays may be obtained for comparison. Computed tomography images may be obtained in the acute setting to further determine congruity of the DRUJ joint. Additionally, magnetic resonance imagery or arthrogram can evaluate TFCC pathology and DRUJ disruption but are not routinely obtained.

The patient should be examined for any additional injuries. After a thorough neurovascular exam and evaluation of forearm compartments, reduction under adequate pain control or sedation should be performed in the emergency department to restore gross alignment. After forearm reduction, instability is determined by increased translation of the distal radius relative to the ulnar head during passive manipulation as the forearm is in neutral position. Increased translation can vary with supination and pronation of the forearm depending on stabilizers injured. Examination is difficult with forearm fractures and must be performed again after the fracture is reduced and stabilized [13]. The patient should then be placed in a well-padded splint and future surgical intervention should be discussed and arranged.

Treatment

Historically, non-operative treatment has been associated with poor results in adults. In 1957, Hughston of the Piedmont Orthopedic Society presented a case series of 41 patients with Galeazzi fractures. He reported unsatisfactory results in 38 patients (92 %) treated with closed reduction and immobilization [21].

In 1975, Mikic [7] reported on 125 patients with classic Galeazzi fractures. Closed reduction and immobilization was performed in 46 patients, including 12 children and 34 adults. Of these treated non-operatively, 80 % of adults had poor results, including patient dissatisfaction, pain, deformity, shortening, or limitation of pronation or supination [7]. Reckling and Peltier [8] reported treatment of Galeazzi lesions in 43 skeletally mature patients. All 17 patients treated with immediate open reduction, internal fixation, and immobilization had a good result with full return of forearm range of motion. Of the 11 patients treated with closed reduction and plaster cast immobilization, 4 patients had fair results, 7 had poor results, and all had restricted pronation and supination [8].

Hughston [21] described four factors as the major causes of loss of reduction. The weight of the hand creates a strong displacing force on the distal radial fragment. This force increases risk for malalignment at the fracture site and subluxation of the DRUJ [21]. The intact pronator quadratus rotates the distal radial fragment toward the ulna, proximal, and volar. The brachioradialis acts to pull the distal radial fragment proximally. Finally, the abductor pollicis longus and extensor pollicis brevis muscles create a shortening deforming force [21].

The Galeazzi fracture-dislocation soon became known as a fracture of necessity, referring to the need for surgical treatment for optimal results. Other eponyms include the Piedmont fracture, the reverse Monteggia fracture, and the Darrach–Hughston–Milch fracture [3, 10]. Misdiagnosis can lead to disabling complications such as DRUJ instability, malunion, limited forearm range of motion, chronic wrist pain, and osteoarthritis.

Currently, open reduction and internal fixation is considered the standard of care for most adult patients with Galeazzi fractures. Anatomic reduction and stable fixation of the radius fracture with assessment and repair of DRUJ instability is essential for favorable outcomes.

Plate fixation is the preferred method for radial fixation and is best achieved with a dynamic compression plate applied through a volar approach [6, 9, 13]. Anatomic reduction of the radial fracture and restoration of the radial bow is important to establish a concentric and stable reduction of the DRUJ [3]. After the radial fracture has been fixed and reduction of the DRUJ confirmed, stability should be tested throughout forearm rotation. Dorsally directed manual stress is applied to the DRUJ in an attempt to dorsally translate the ulnar head out of the sigmoid notch [6, 13]. Translation can be compared to the contralateral side as laxity can vary in patients under anesthesia. If stable, the patient can be placed in an above elbow splint in neutral to supination.

A reduced but unstable DRUJ can be temporarily transfixed with two K-wires, inserted percutaneously just proximal to the sigmoid notch with the forearm neutral to slightly supination. These K-wires are left in place for 4–6 weeks to maintain congruency during soft tissue healing [3, 6, 9, 10]. If the DRUJ is irreducible after fixation of the radius, interposition of soft tissue must be considered with the extensor carpi ulnaris tendon documented as the most common [18, 22]. TFCC repair is typically performed with direct visualization through a dorsal approach, using drill holes or suture anchor technique [23]. If there is an ulnar styloid fracture, fixation with K-wires or a tension-band technique can increase stability due to attachments of the TFCC ligaments to the ulnar styloid [6].

Complications

Galeazzi fractures have many of the same complications as all forearm fractures, including nerve compression, tendon entrapment, nonunion, delayed union, malunion, and infection [6]. The most common and devastating complication includes angulation at the fracture site and subluxation or dislocation of the DRUJ, typically from misdiagnosis or inappropriate treatment [6, 13].

Again, Hughston in 1957 [21] believed that the 92 % unsatisfactory results of conservative treatment were due to most physicians' lack of knowledge of the deforming forces during conservative management. "The rareness of this fracture, therefore, our unfamiliarity with it, accounts for our lack of knowledge of its complex aspects." [21]

With 125 patients, Mikic [7] encountered subluxation or dislocation with inadequate radial reduction and fixation. Mikic stated that "when open reduction and internal fixation of the radius, the DRUJ should always be tested for stability and in cases where it is unstable obviously something must be done." [7] Delayed treatment only increases risks for nonunion, recurrent dislocation and infection, and chronic pain [3].

In patients with nonunion or malunion after late presentation, restoring radial length and DRUJ congruity may be possible with a radial osteotomy with plating and bone grafting [3, 6]. Otherwise, salvage procedures can be performed to decrease pain and increase range of motion associated with chronic DRUJ instability. These salvage techniques include the Darrach procedure, hemiresection arthroplasty, Sauve–Kapandji procedure, or implant arthroplasty [6, 13].

Summary

A Galeazzi fracture-dislocation, known as a "fracture of necessity," is an unstable injury that requires recognition, open reduction and internal fixation to achieve satisfactory outcomes. Complications are associated with unrecognized DRUJ injury or incomplete reduction and stabilization such as chronic DRUJ pain and limited forearm and wrist range of motion. With fracture of the radial shaft, a surgeon must have a high suspicion of DRUJ instability and perform a thorough examination after radial fixation. Anatomical fixation of the radius fracture and DRUJ stabilization reduce the need of future salvage procedures associated with a missed or inadequately treated Galeazzi fracture-dislocation.

References

1. Reckling FW. Unstable fracture-dislocations of the forearm (Monteggia and Galeazzi lesions). J Bone Joint Surg Am. 1982;64(6):857–63.
2. Macule Beneyto F, Arandes Renu JM, Ferreres Claramunt A, Ramon SR. Treatment of Galeazzi fracture-dislocations. J Trauma. 1994;36(3):352–5.

3. Giannoulis FS, Sotereanos DG. Galeazzi fractures and dislocations. Hand Clin. 2007;23(2):153–63. v.

4. Cooper A. Simple fracture of the radius and dislocation of the ulna. In: Cooper A, editor. A treatise on dislocations, and on fractures of the joints. London: Longman; 1825. p. 470–6.

5. Galeazzi R. Di una particolare sindrome traumatica dello scheletro dell 'avambraccio. Atti e memorie della Societa'lombarda di chirurgia. 1934;2:663–6.

6. Atesok KI, Jupiter JB, Weiss AP. Galeazzi fracture. J Am Acad Orthop Surg. 2011;19(10):623–33.

7. Mikic ZD. Galeazzi fracture-dislocations. J Bone Joint Surg Am. 1975;57(8):1071–80.

8. Reckling FW, Peltier LF. Riccardo Galeazzi and Galeazzi's Fracture. Surgery. 1965;58:453–9.

9. Rettig ME, Raskin KB. Galeazzi fracture-dislocation: a new treatment-oriented classification. J Hand Surg Am. 2001;26(2):228–35.

10. Sebastin SJ, Chung KC. A historical report on Riccardo Galeazzi and the management of Galeazzi fractures. J Hand Surg Am. 2010;35(11):1870–7.

11. Huang JI, Hanel DP. Anatomy and biomechanics of the distal radioulnar joint. Hand Clin. 2012;28(2):157–63.

12. Palmer AK, Werner FW. The triangular fibrocartilage complex of the wrist–anatomy and function. J Hand Surg Am. 1981;6(2):153–62.

13. Ruchelsman DE, Raskin KB, Rettig ME. Galeazzi fracture-dislocations. In: Slutsky DJ, Osterman AL, editors. Fractures and injuries of the distal radius and carpus. Philadelphia: Saunders/Elsevier; 2009. p. 231–9.

14. Palmer AK, Werner FW. Biomechanics of the distal radioulnar joint. Clin Orthop Relat Res. 1984;187:26–35.

15. Gofton WT, Gordon KD, Dunning CE, Johnson JA, King GJ. Soft-tissue stabilizers of the distal radioulnar joint: an in vitro kinematic study. J Hand Surg Am. 2004;29(3):423–31.

16. Dameron Jr TB. Traumatic dislocation of the distal radio-ulnar joint. Clin Orthop Relat Res. 1972;83:55–63.

17. Walsh HP, McLaren CA, Owen R. Galeazzi fractures in children. J Bone Joint Surg Br. 1987;69(5):730–3.

18. Carlsen BT, Dennison DG, Moran SL. Acute dislocations of the distal radioulnar joint and distal ulna fractures. Hand Clin. 2010;26(4):503–16.

19. Loredo RA, Sorge DG, Garcia G. Radiographic evaluation of the wrist: a vanishing art. Semin Roentgenol. 2005;40(3):248–89.

20. Schneiderman G, Meldrum RD, Bloebaum RD, Tarr R, Sarmiento A. The interosseous membrane of the forearm: structure and its role in Galeazzi fractures. J Trauma. 1993;35(6):879–85.

21. Hughston JC. Fracture of the distal radial shaft; mistakes in management. J Bone Joint Surg Am. 1957;39-A(2):249–64; passim.

22. Bruckner JD, Lichtman DM, Alexander AH. Complex dislocations of the distal radioulnar joint. Recognition and management. Clin Orthop Relat Res. 1992;275:90–103.

23. Trumble TE, Culp RW, Hanel DP, Geissler WB, Berger RA. Intra-articular fractures of the distal aspect of the radius. Instr Course Lect. 1999;48:465–80.

Chapter 16
Distal Radius Fractures: A Clinical Casebook

Pediatric Metaphyseal Fracture Open Reduction and Internal Fixation

Jamie Cowan and Jeffrey N. Lawton

Case History

A 15-year-old right-handed male sustained a hyperextension injury to his left wrist while playing hockey. The injury occurred when he collided with another player. He experienced immediate wrist pain and reports feeling "a large pop" in his wrist. He presented to a local Emergency Department where radiographs revealed a bicortical transverse fracture of the distal radial metaphysis (Fig. 16.1) with approximately 14° of dorsal angulation of the distal fracture fragment. There was comminution of the dorsal cortex and the radial fracture line extended obliquely to within 5 mm of the distal radial physis. There was also an associated ulnar styloid fracture. He denied prior history of significant injury or surgery to the left wrist.

After discussing the risks and benefits of both nonoperative and surgical management, the patient and his parents elected to proceed with distal radius open reduction and internal fixation with

J. Cowan, MD (✉) • J.N. Lawton, MD
Department of Orthopaedic Surgery, University of Michigan Health System, A. Alfred Taubman Health Care Center, Floor 2, Reception: B, 2912 Taubman Center, 1500 East Medical Center Drive, Ann Arbor, MI 48109-5328, USA
e-mail: cowanj@med.umich.edu

© Springer International Publishing Switzerland 2016   201
J.N. Lawton (ed.), *Distal Radius Fractures*,
DOI 10.1007/978-3-319-27489-8_16

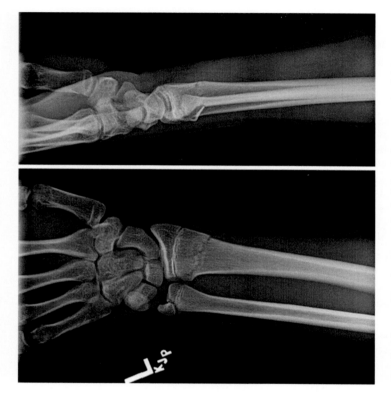

Fig. 16.1 Initial radiographs of a 15-year-old male who sustained a left wrist hyperextension injury

possible ulnar styloid fixation depending on the stability of the DRUJ after addressing the radius fracture. The patient was taken to the operating room 3 days after his injury. The distal radius was approached through flexor carpi radialis (FCR) tendon sheath and the pronator quadratus was elevated off of the radius, proximally. However, care was taken to avoid injury by dissection in the area of the physis and perichondrium. Using a volar locking distal radius plate, the fracture was reduced and stabilized with a combination of locking screws traversing the Thurston-Holland metaphyseal fragment and non-locking screws, proximally. After achieving anatomic reduction of the radius, evaluation of the DRUJ revealed asymmetric instability. Consequently the fracture at the base of the ulna styloid was addressed through a separate incision. The ulna fracture was anatomically reduced and stabilized with a single 0.045-inch Kirschner wire and FiberWire (Arthrex; Naples, Florida) suture in cerclage technique. The DRUJ was then reevaluated and stability had been achieved. The pronator quadratus was repaired, subcutaneous tissue and skin were closed, and the patient was placed in a well-padded long-arm splint in supination for 2 weeks.

At his clinic appointment approximately 6 weeks after surgery, the patient denied any pain in the left wrist. Examination revealed no tenderness to palpation and full active range of motion in all planes compared with the contralateral side. The patient gradually increased activity as tolerated and by approximately 12 weeks after surgery he had returned to his pre-operative level of activity without restriction—including a return to hockey. His most recent radiographs, at final follow-up, approximately 10 months after surgery showed healed distal radius and ulnar styloid fractures with appropriate alignment (Fig. 16.2).

Discussion

Distal radius fractures, particularly metaphyseal fractures, are common injuries in pediatric populations [1–4]. In fact, distal forearm fractures are becoming more common, with hypothesized causes including increased physical activity, increased childhood

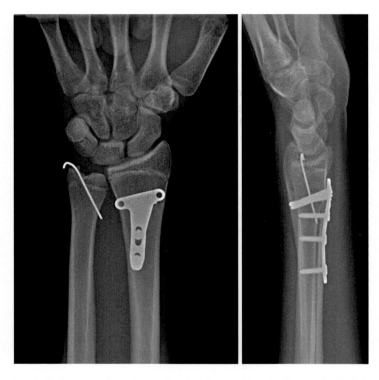

Fig. 16.2 Postoperative radiographs of a 15-year-old male who sustained a left wrist hyperextension injury

obesity, changing dietary habits, and decreased bone density [5–7]. Most of these injuries may be treated with nonoperative management [8]. Thorough clinical evaluation with regular follow-up, and in the case of operative intervention, meticulous surgical technique, must be employed when caring for injuries about the physes of growing children. Decisions regarding treatment are made taking into account deformity and the amount of growth remaining/ potential for remodeling—recognizing the differences in skeletal maturity between boys and girls. The distal radial physis accounts for up to 80 % of longitudinal growth of the radius and allows for significant remodeling potential following distal radius fractures [9].

In addition to careful radiographic evaluation of physeal involvement, thorough neurovascular assessment and documentation is always indicated in the setting of acute trauma. This may be particularly important for completely displaced fractures in which satisfactory closed reduction cannot be obtained. For example, periosteum or pronator quadratus entrapment can prevent satisfactory closed reduction and multiple reduction attempts may results in further physeal injury, cumulative soft-tissue trauma, neuropraxia, increased compartment pressures, risks of conscious sedation, and increased cost [9–11].

While there is no common or prognostically useful classification system for pediatric distal radius fractures, it is helpful to consider these injuries with respect to the characteristics used to describe any pediatric fracture: location, displacement, angulation, physeal involvement, articular involvement, and mechanism of injury [12].

Non-Displaced and Minimally Displaced Fractures

Non-displaced, unicortical, "incomplete" compression injuries to the distal radial metaphysis are frequently referred to as torus, unicortical, or "buckle" fractures. These inherently stable injuries are due to plastic deformation or a fracture at the area of transition between woven metaphyseal bone and lamellar diaphyseal bone [13, 14]. Such fractures usually result from relatively low-energy falls [15].

Two randomized studies that compared treatment of distal radius torus fractures with either casts or removable splints found no differences in outcomes or complications [13, 16]. One of these studies also found that patients randomized to removable splints fared better with activities of daily living and bathing [16]. West et al. [17] randomized patients to either a below-elbow plaster cast or a soft bandage. This study found no differences in healing or complications, but found that patients treated with only a soft bandage demonstrated significantly greater wrist range of motion at 4 weeks after injury. Symons et al. [18] found no difference in outcome depending on whether splints were removed at clinical follow-up or at home.

Minimally displaced fractures of the distal radius may be treated nonoperatively even if they are complete bicortical fractures. This is due to the capacity for remodeling of skeletally immature bone [10, 19]. The focus of treatment is maintenance of adequate alignment and prevention of further displacement. A randomized controlled trial by Boutis et al. [19] compared short-arm fiberglass casts with prefabricated wrist splints for the treatment of minimally angulated (≤15° in the sagittal plane) and minimally displaced (≤5 mm translation in the frontal plane) distal radial metaphyseal fractures. The authors found no differences between groups in range of motion, grip strength, pain, or fracture angulation. Although all parents in the study were satisfied with treatment, both patients and parents reported a preference for splinting over casting.

In summary, torus and minimally displaced distal radius fractures are stable injuries that tend to do well even without long-term immobilization or follow-up. These fractures do not require surgical intervention by an orthopedic surgeon and may be safely managed by general pediatricians.

Displaced Fractures

Treatment of significantly displaced distal radius fractures remains somewhat controversial. Most physicians advocate for initial management by closed reduction, under a local anesthetic hematoma block or conscious sedation, and immobilization. Regardless of the mechanism of injury, reduction can often be achieved by exaggeration of the deformity, longitudinal traction, and restoration of anatomical alignment [15]. Although not specific for fractures of the distal radius, two prospective randomized controlled trials studies found that displaced distal forearm fractures requiring reduction may be adequately treated with either short-arm or long-arm casts [20, 21]. One of these studies showed significantly higher cast indices among fractures in which reduction was lost, highlighting the importance of proper cast-application technique [21]. Immobilization is generally required for 4–6 weeks following such injuries.

Miller et al. [22] compared closed reduction and cast immobilization to closed reduction, percutaneous pin fixation, and cast immobilization in patients older than 10 years with distal radius fractures that were completely displaced or had greater than 30° of dorsal angulation. There were no significant differences in complication rates, cost, or long-term results between groups. Thirty-nine percent of patients treated with casting required remanipulation due to loss of reduction. While there were no instances of loss of reduction in the group treated with pin fixation, 38 % of patients had pin-related complications such as infection, migration, or tendon irritation.

The risk of redisplacement following closed reduction of displaced distal radius and forearm fractures varies from approximately 9–39 % [8, 22–29]. Mazzini et al. [3] reviewed this subject, as well as various casting indices, and described factors leading to loss of reduction as either fracture-related, surgeon-related, or patient-related (Table 16.1). Factors associated with redisplacement include initial displacement, fracture obliquity, direction of angulation, quality of initial reduction, experience of the individual performing the reduction [8, 23, 25, 26, 29]. Given these numerous contributing factors and relatively high rates of displacement, frequent clinical follow-up with serial radiographic evaluation is mandatory when treating displaced distal radius fractures nonoperatively.

However there are varying opinions as to what constitutes "acceptable" alignment of distal radius fractures. For example, Bae et al. [30] described acceptable criteria as 10° of frontal plane angulation, 20–25° of sagittal plane angulation, and no malrotation if more than 5 years of growth remain. Noonan and Price [31] define acceptable criteria as completed displacement, 15° of angulation, and 45° of malrotation in patients under 9 years old; 15° of angulation and 15° of malrotation in patients over 9 years old, and complete bayonet apposition and 20° of angulation in patients with no more than 2 years of growth remaining. Other indications for surgical treatment of distal radius fractures may include irre-

Table 16.1 Factors leading to loss of reduction of pediatric distal forearm and radius fractures (adapted from Mazzini et al. [3])

Fracture-related factors	Initial displacement
	Fracture location
	Fracture obliquity
	Proximity to physis
	Radius and ulna fractures at the same level
Surgeon-related factors	Inadequate initial closed reduction
	Poor casting technique
Patient-related factors	Resolution of soft tissue swelling
	Muscle atrophy
	Noncompliance with activity restrictions

ducible fractures, open fractures, floating elbow injuries, polytrauma, neurovascular compromise, or soft tissue injury precluding adequate immobilization [9]. Despite these guidelines, studies have shown good results with closed reduction of significantly displaced distal radius fractures. Cannata et al. [32] reviewed 157 distal forearm physeal fractures, 73 of which were moderately or severely displaced, at an average of 25.5 years. All injuries were treated with closed reduction and immobilization. They found no symptoms or functional problems in patients with less than 1 cm of radioulnar length discrepancy. Crawford et al. [33] treated 51 closed, shorted, overriding distal radial metaphyseal fractures in patients under 10 years old with casting in situ without analgesia, sedation, or reduction. At a minimum of 1 year after injury, all patients achieved painless clinical and radiographic union, full wrist range of motion, good grip strength, and complete satisfaction among parents/guardians.

Open reduction and volar plating may be appropriate for displaced metaphyseal fractures when pinning may be difficult due to fracture pattern, adequate closed reduction cannot be achieved, or in patients with fewer than 2 years of skeletal growth remaining [30]. Additionally, if a metaphyseal fracture extends to the articular surface (as in a Salter-Harris type IV fracture), anatomic reduction usually requires an open approach. The goal of open reduction and internal fixation is anatomic reduction without causing additional injury to the physis, periosteum, or perichondrium. Theoretical advantages of volar plate fixation include anatomic reduction, compression across the fracture site, greater control of fracture fragments, greater mechanical stability, and early range of motion, while theoretical disadvantages include greater surgical dissection, bothersome hardware requiring removal, and superficial scar formation.

There is little high-quality literature regarding volar plate fixation of metaphyseal distal radius fractures in the pediatric population. The technique is similar to the technique used for adults, in which the fracture is approached between the FCR and radial artery. In pediatric patients, meticulous surgical exposure and delicate tissue handling are paramount for avoiding iatrogenic injury to the physis, periosteum, and perichondrium. The perichondrium plays a principal role in endochondral ossification as a source of osteoblasts and endothelial cells, and as a conduit for blood vessels into hypertrophic cartilage [34]. Injury to these tissues puts the patient at risk for subsequent problems with the maturation and development of the growing limb. Based upon the fracture pattern, sometimes it may not be possible to avoid having the plate span the physis/epiphysis. In these cases, the plate may be slightly undercontoured and then secured proximally without screws placed distally — merely laid over the perichondrium/periosteum with a spring plate technique employed.

Conclusions

Fractures of the distal radial metaphysis are common in children of all ages. Despite a wide spectrum of severity of injury, many of these fractures may be treated with closed reduction (if necessary) and immobilization. The quality of the reduction and casting technique are likely more important than the specific type of immobilization. In these cases, serial clinical evaluation and radiographs are indicated to ensure adequate nonoperative management. Although there are not clear prognostic criteria for which of these injuries require operative intervention, factors associated with fracture redisplacement include initial displacement, fracture obliquity, direction of angulation, quality of initial reduction, and the experience of the individual performing the reduction. When surgical management is indicated, basic principles of fracture management should guide the surgeon toward achieving a stable internal fixation construct and successful outcome. Regardless of whether nonoperative or surgical management is ultimately pursued, meticulous technique and a thorough knowledge of pediatric anatomy and bone physiology are crucial for avoiding poor outcomes including permanent deformity or premature physeal closure.

References

1. Bae DS, Howard AW. Distal Radius Fractures: What Is the Evidence? J Pediatr Orthop. 2012;32(2):S128–30.
2. Cheng JC, Shen WY. Limb fracture pattern in different pediatric age groups: a study of 3350 children. J Orthop Trauma. 1993;7(1):15–22.
3. Mazzini JP, Martin JR. Paediatric forearm and distal radius fractures: risk factors and redisplacement – role of casting indices. Int Orthop. 2010;34: 407–12.
4. Ward WT, Rihn JA. The impact of Trauma in an Urban pediatric orthopaedic practice. J Bone Joint Surg Am. 2006;88-A(12):2759–64.
5. Khosla S, Melton LJ, Dekutoski MB, Achenbach SJ, Oberg AL, Riggs BL. Incidence of childhood distal forearm fractures over 30 years: a population-based study. JAMA. 2003;290(11):1479–85.
6. Goulding A, Jones IE, Taylor RW, Williams SM, Manning PJ. Bone mineral density and body composition in boys with distal forearm fractures: a dual-energy x-ray absorptiometry study. J Pediatr. 2001;139(4):509–15.
7. Nellans KW, Kowalski E, Chung KC. The epidemiology of distal radius fractures. Hand Clin. 2012;28(2):113–25.
8. Proctor MT, Moore DJ, Paterson JM. Redisplacement after manipulation of distal radial fractures in children. J Bone Joint Surg Br. 1993;75-B(3): 453–4.
9. Bae DS, Waters PM. Pediatric distal radius fractures and triangular fibrocartilage complex injuries. Hand Clin. 2006;22(1):43–53.
10. Do TT, Strub WM, Foad SL, Mehlman CT, Crawford AH. Reduction versus remodeling in pediatric distal forearm fractures: a preliminary cost analysis. J Pediatr Orthop Part B. 2003;12(2):109–15.
11. Holmes JR, Louis DL. Entrapment of pronator quadratus in pediatric distal radius fractures: recognition and treatment. J Pediatr Orthop. 1994;14(4): 498–500.
12. Dolan M, Waters PM. Fractures and dislocations of the forearm, wrist, and hand. In: Green NE, Swiontkowski MF, editors. Skeletal Trauma in children. 4th ed. Philadelphia, PA: Elsevier; 2009.

13. Davidson JS, Brown DJ, Barnes SN, Bruce CE. Simple treatment for torus fractures of the distal radius. J Bone Joint Surg Br. 2001;83-B(8):1173–5.
14. Light TR, Ogden DA, Ogden JA. The anatomy of metaphyseal torus fractures. Clin Orthop Relat Res. 1984;188:103–11.
15. Upper extremity injuries. In: Herring JA, editor. Tachdjian's pediatric orthopaedics. 5th ed. Philadelphia, PA: Elsevier; 2014.
16. Plint AC, Perry JJ, Correll R, Gaboury I, Lawton L. A randomized, controlled trial of removable splinting versus casting for wrist buckle fractures in children. Pediatrics. 2006;117(3):691–7.
17. West S, Andrews J, Bebbington A, Ennis O, Alderman P. Buckle fractures of the distal radius are safely treated in a soft bandage. J Pediatr Orthop. 2005;25(3):322–5.
18. Symons S, Rowsell M, Bhowal B, Dias JJ. Hospital versus home management of children with buckle fractures of the distal radius. J Bone Joint Surg Br. 2001;83-B(4):556–60.
19. Boutis K, Willan A, Babyn P, Goeree R, Howard A. Cast versus splint in children with minimally angulated fractures of the distal radius: a randomized controlled trial. CMAJ. 2010;182(14):1507–12.
20. Bohm ER, Bubbar V, Hing KY, Dzus A. Above and below-the-elbow plaster casts for distal forearm fractures in children. J Bone Joint Surg Am. 2006;88-A(1):1–8.
21. Webb GR, Galpin RD, Armstrong DG. Comparison of short and long arm plaster casts for displaced fractures in the distal third of the forearm in children. J Bone Joint Surg Am. 2006;88-A(1):9–17.
22. Miller BS, Taylor B, Widmann RF, Bae DS, Snyder BD, Waters PM. Cast immobilization versus percutaneous pin fixation of displaced distal radius fractures in children. J Pediatr Orthop. 2005;25(4):490–4.
23. Alemdaroglu KB, Iltar S, Cimen O, Uysal M, Alagoz E, Atlihan D. Risk factors in redisplacement of distal radial fractures in children. J Bone Joint Surg Am. 2008;90(6):1224–30.
24. Gibbons CL, Woods DA, Pailthorpe C, Carr AJ, Worlock P. The management of isolated distal radius fractures in children. J Pediatr Orthop. 1994;14(2):207–10.
25. Haddad FS, Williams RL. Forearm fractures in children: avoiding redisplacement. Injury. 1995;26(10):691–2.
26. Mani GV, Hui PW, Cheng JC. Translation of the radius as a predictor of outcome in distal radial fractures of children. J Bone Joint Surg Br. 1993;75-B(5):808–11.
27. McLauchlan GJ, Cowan B, Annan IH, Robb JE. Management of completely displaced metaphyseal fractures of the distal radius in children. J Bone Joint Surg Br. 2002;84-B(3):413–7.
28. McQuinn AG, Jaarsma RL. Risk factors for redisplacement of pediatric distal forearm and distal radius fractures. J Pediatr Orthop. 2012;32(7):687–92.
29. Zamzam MM, Khoshhal KI. Displaced fracture of the distal radius in children: factors responsible for redisplacement after closed reduction. J Bone Joint Surg Br. 2005;87-B(6):841–3.

30. Bae DS. Pediatric distal radius and forearm fractures. J Hand Surg Am. 2008;33(10):1911–23.
31. Noonan KJ, Price CT. Forearm and distal radius fractures in children. JAAOS. 1998;6(3):146–56.
32. Cannata G, De Maio F, Mancini F, Ippolito E. Physeal fractures of the distal radius and Ulna: long-term prognosis. J Orthop Trauma. 2003;17(3):172–9.
33. Crawford SN, Lee LS, Izuka BH. Closed treatment of overriding distal radial fractures without reduction in children. J Bone Joint Surg Am. 2012;94(3):246–52.
34. Colnot C, Lu C, Hu D, Helms JA. Distinguishing the contributions of the perichondrium, cartilage, and vascular endothelium to skeletal development. Dev Biol. 2004;269(1):55–69.

Chapter 17
Loss of Fixation in Distal Radius Fractures

Michael B. Geary and John C. Elfar

Case Presentation

A 59-year-old right-hand dominant male was involved in a motorcycle collision, in which he collided with a car while traveling approximately 40 miles per hour. He suffered multiple injuries, including a closed-head injury and pelvic fractures, along with an intraarticular comminuted volar Barton's distal radius fracture (Fig. 17.1a, b). During the initial hospital admission, after his pelvic injuries were stabilized, he was taken to surgery for operative fixation of his distal radius fracture. Volar plate fixation was selected and placed (Fig. 17.1c, d), though there was some concern

M.B. Geary, MD
University of Rochester School of Medicine and Dentistry Center for Musculoskeletal Research, Rochester, NY 14642, USA
e-mail: Michael_Geary@urmc.rochester.edu

J.C. Elfar, MD (✉)
University of Rochester School of Medicine and Dentistry Center for Musculoskeletal Research, Rochester, NY 14642, USA

Department of Orthopaedic Surgery, Hand and Upper Extremity and Sports Medicine, University of Rochester Medical Center, Rochester, NY 14642, USA
e-mail: openelfar@gmail.com

© Springer International Publishing Switzerland 2016
J.N. Lawton (ed.), *Distal Radius Fractures*,
DOI 10.1007/978-3-319-27489-8_17

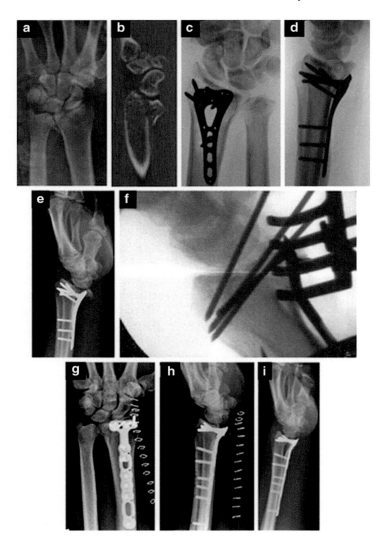

Fig. 17.1 Loss of fixation after volar plate fixation of volar shearing distal radius fracture. (**a**) AP radiograph after initial closed reduction. (**b**) Lateral radiograph demonstrating the intraarticular fracture pattern and the volar shearing fragment. (**c**) AP radiograph of the initial fixation showing volar plate fixation with extra-articular screw placement. (**d**) Lateral radiograph of the

over fixation of the distal volar fragment, appreciated best on the lateral radiograph. Within one week following the initial plate fixation, catastrophic loss of fixation was evident (Fig. 17.1e). Though the initial plate buttressed and fixed some of the fragments of the unstable volar lip of the distal radius, excessive motion during immobilization, in addition to poor overall fixation, resulted in dislocation of the carpus anterior to the plate-screw construct (Fig. 17.1e). Revision surgery was undertaken, and the decision was made to use a volar approach with removal of the hardware and placement of a new volar plate on the volar lip, with screws directed retrograde to support the volar lip while fixing the volar lip fragment in place. During the placement of this second plate, a pin was strategically placed through the lunate into the dorsal lip of the radius to maintain reduction and to relieve pressure from the volar surface of the distal radius (Fig. 17.1f). Excellent fixation was achieved in this revision surgery (Fig. 17.1g, h), and the patient healed without event (Fig. 17.1i). Final range of motion (ROM) was approximately 50° in flexion and extension.

Background and Review of the Literature

When confronted with fractures of the distal radius, the treating orthopedist should aim to achieve the best possible anatomic reduction, while minimizing the risk of short- and long-term complications. Loss of fracture fixation, or loss of reduction, is one such complication, and it is important to understand the ways in which reduction can be lost, along with the risk factors that

Fig. 17.1 (continued) initial volar plate fixation. (**e**) Lateral radiograph taken one week after initial fixation, demonstrating loss of fixation of the distal volar fragment and dislocation of the carpus anterior to the plate-screw construct. (**f**) Lateral radiograph during revision surgery, showing temporary pinning of the lunate to the dorsal lip of the distal radius. (**g**) AP radiograph of revision volar plate fixation. (**h**) Lateral radiograph of the revision volar plate fixation. (**i**) Lateral radiograph at 7 months followup after revision surgery, demonstrating adequate fracture healing and no recurrent loss of fixation

predispose certain patients and fracture patterns to this complication. Further, one must be equipped to manage the loss of fixation, and to determine whether further surgical intervention is warranted, or if the malalignment can be managed conservatively. For example, in young, active patients, it is often worthwhile to intervene to achieve a more anatomic reduction, whereas elderly patients with lower functional demands may be able to tolerate some loss of fixation [1–3].

There are a variety of ways in which reduction can be lost, and there is a range of functional consequences associated with the radiographic changes [4]. In his review of malunited distal radius fractures, Graham described and popularized five common radiographic parameters used to evaluate the distal radius: radial inclination, radial length, ulnar variance, radial tilt, and radial shift [5]. Among the changes, ulnar variance and radial tilt (referred to more often as dorsal tilt) are most frequently reported in outcomes studies of different fixation methods for distal radius fractures (Fig. 17.2). Fixation is also susceptible to failure at the lunate facet in volar shearing-type fractures; small fragments, in particular, can be challenging, since there is limited bone for distal screw purchase. Additionally, bulky plates in this area potentially compromise the digital flexors. In general, risk factors for loss of fixation include older age, dorsal angulation greater than 20°, dorsal comminution, intraarticular fracture patterns, and associated ulna fractures [6, 7].

Ulnar positive variance, referred to also as radial shortening, occurs when the articular surface of the ulna projects more distal than radius, occurring secondary to settling of the distal fragment. Some believe that radial shortening may be due to inappropriate positioning of the distal screws in a volar plate construct relative to the subchondral bone. This understanding suggests that screws should be placed directly supporting the subchondral bone, so as to prevent fracture fragments from settling [8–10]. In a cadaveric study of extra-articular distal radius fractures (AO type A3), screws placed more than 4 mm proximal to the subchondral bone had a 73.9 % increase in radial shortening compared to those placed as close to the subchondral zone as possible (1.38 mm vs. 0.36 mm) [11]. It is unclear whether or not cadaveric studies represent a true recapitulation of clinical experience, for subchondral bone screw

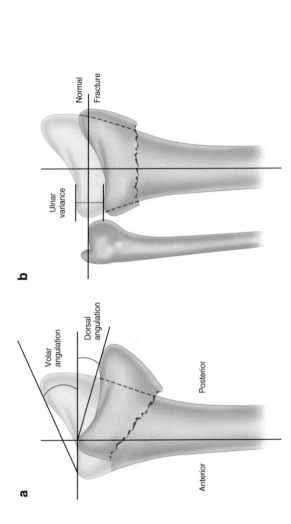

Fig. 17.2 Dorsal angulation and ulnar variance. (**a**) Lateral schematic demonstrating dorsal angulation of the distal radius fragment. The normal border of the distal radius is indicated by the dotted line. (**b**) Distal radius fracture settling demonstrating positive ulnar variance. The distal fragment settles proximally and causes relative lengthening of the ulna

placement may paradoxically raise the risk of catastrophic screw cutout into the joint in patients with exceedingly fragile bone — thus trading a minor complication for a major one.

The functional consequences of positive ulnar variance are many. Relative shortening of the radius increases the load on the ulna, leading to decreased ROM, wrist pain, loss of grip strength, and loss of forearm rotation [12–15]. In studies comparing radiographic changes to subjective outcomes, radial shortening of greater than 2 mm has been shown to be a strong predictor of poor function and low satisfaction [16–19]. As such, full radial length may be critical to achieving satisfactory long-term results.

Dorsal tilt is the angle between the articular surface of the distal radius and a line perpendicular to the long axis of the radius on the lateral radiographs. Dorsal tilt of distal radius fractures occurs from falls on the extended wrist, and may recur after initial reduction and fixation. After radial shortening, dorsal tilt is thought to be the next most significant predictor of poor clinical outcomes [20] as it alters the mechanics of the wrist and can shift more of the load onto the ulna. In a biomechanical study, as the angulation of the distal radial fragment increased from 10° of palmar tilt (normal) to 45° of dorsal tilt, the load through the ulna increased from 21 % to 67 % of the total load across the wrist [17]. These changes have been associated with pain, decreases in grip strength, and difficulties with activities of daily living [21–23]. With dorsal tilt greater than 10°, DASH scores [24] have been shown to increase by 10.5 points when compared to fractures with normal dorsal angulation [25]. This was true even when patients were controlled for age, sex, and treatment types. Dorsal tilt predicts outcomes, and rigid fixation to preserve the normal palmar tilt of the distal radius seems critical, and loss of fixation of this parameter may independently result in poorer outcomes.

The lunate facet comprises the ulnar side of the articular surface of the distal radius, and more comminuted fracture patterns may leave small fragments in this region difficult to fix. Radiographic evaluation of the lunate facet is best achieved with the tangential lateral radiograph [26]. Some criticism of volar plate design has been mounted over the utility of this plate in certain types of distal radius fractures, specifically AO type B3.2

and B3.3 fractures where there may not be a distal volar-lunate extension to allow adequate fixation of these fragments [27]. Among the most significant predictors of loss of lunate facet fixation is the length of volar cortex available to accept hardware, as measured from the articular margin to the fracture line [28]. In a study of 52 volar shearing distal radius fractures treated with volar plates, the 7 fractures that lost fixation were all AO type B3.3 fractures, and multivariate logistic regression revealed that a critical 15 mm of volar cortex available to accept hardware significantly decreased the risk for loss of reduction. In cases where less than 15 mm is available, the authors recommended additional means of fixation [28].

Having provided an overview of the ways that fixation may be lost, it is important now to examine the different treatment modalities and the available literature on loss of reduction with the most common approaches for fixation.

Loss of Fixation After Percutaneous Pinning

Among fixation methods for distal radius fractures, percutaneous pinning offers the benefit of being minimally invasive and inexpensive relative to other fixation options. While percutaneous pinning can be used for two- and three-part fractures, it is less effective in fractures with severe comminution or articular shearing [29]. There is concern over how reliably percutaneous pinning can maintain fracture reduction, and whether the distal fragment settles during the initial postoperative period [30–33]. In a review of 85 displaced, extra-articular fractures (AO type A2.2 or A3) treated with percutaneous pinning, Yang et al. reported early fracture collapse as indicated by increasing ulnar variance, along with increasing dorsal tilt [34]. This is consistent with other studies of percutaneous pinning for extra-articular fractures [35, 36]. Kennedy et al. reviewed 72 cases of dorsally angulated, AO type A3 fractures managed with percutaneous pinning [37]. At 6-weeks post-fixation, 56.8 % of cases had radial shortening of 2 mm or more. In some cases, an additional 1 or 2 distal radius-ulnar pins may be added through the subchondral bone for extra support, and studies suggest that this may help to avoid the development of positive ulnar variance [38].

Dorsal angulation after percutaneous pinning can also be a source of fixation failure. In their retrospective review of 55 cases of distal radius fractures treated with percutaneous pinning, 4 patients lost 5° or more of volar tilt and became dorsally angulated [29]. Of the 10 patients who failed to achieve adequate reduction in a study by Barton et al., only one had failure to correct dorsal angulation; the other losses were all cases of radial shortening [35].

Nonetheless, percutaneous pinning for distal radius fractures remains an important tool. Some degree of radial shortening and dorsal angulation has been reported after surgery, which does represent failure of fixation in the strictest sense; but may remain clinically acceptable.

Loss of Fixation After Volar Plating

Volar plating has become increasingly popular for the management of distal radius fractures due to the relatively straightforward approach from the palmar side and the added strength and stability that plating can provide. Further, in fractures with high degrees of comminution, the fixed-angle construct and locked screws improve the anatomic healing potential of the metaphyseal fragments. Perhaps the best reason for volar plate fixation is the knowledge that with a relatively unobtrusive location of hardware beneath the pronator quadratus,j the distal radius is supported so rigidly that early finger and wrist range motion can be initiated.

Studies of radiographic outcomes with volar plating for distal radius fractures report variable rates of loss of fixation. Unlike percutaneous pinning, plate fixation can be used for fractures with high degrees of comminution, which can be an independent predictor of loss of fixation. In Rozental and Blazer's review of 41 patients with dorsally displaced, comminuted distal radius fractures treated with volar plates, the four cases of loss of fixation were all fractures with high degrees of dorsal comminution; two

AO type A3, one type C2, and one type C3 [39]. Notably, two of the fixation failures presented with excessive dorsal angulation, and two presented with loss of adequate fixation at the lunate facet. However, despite the loss of reduction, none of the patients required further intervention and all were satisfied with their outcomes. These failure and satisfaction rates are similar to those reported by Gogna et al. in their study of 33 patients with dorsally comminuted fractures treated with volar locked plates [40]. In this series, the authors describe three cases where fixation was lost, all presenting with collapse and dorsal tilt. The first case was an example of a missed distal radio-ulnar joint (DRUJ) injury, emphasizing the importance of assessing the integrity of the DRUJ in all fractures of the distal radius. The other two failures were in AO type C3 fractures, and both patients were satisfied with their subjective outcomes and accepted deformity without revision surgery. In these studies and others, high degrees of dorsal comminution were associated with loss of fixation [41].

With greater comminution, there may be cases where the lunate facet is difficult to fix with the volar plate, increasing the risk for loss of fixation. In a case series of seven patients with volar shearing fractures of the distal radius (AO type B3), every case lost reduction of the volar lunate facet [42]. Five of the seven were symptomatic and required revision surgery. This fracture pattern, in particular, presents a challenge for fixation with volar plating alone (see Chap. 8).

Loss of Fixation After Dorsal Plating

Dorsal plate fixation for distal radius fractures is occasionally used due to the improved visualization of the articular surface offered by the dorsal approach, and the option it allows for placement of a dorsal buttress to the internal fixation [43, 44]. While used less often than volar plating, surgeon preference and fracture patterns may favor dorsal over volar plating in certain instances. The dorsal plate lies directly over the portion of the fracture most commonly comminuted. It therefore has the benefit of addressing the area of greatest injury and avoids the detriments of placing the plate directly beneath critically important and fragile flexor tendons. Rates of tendon rupture after dorsal hardware placement are high [45]. However, the dorsal approach, more than any other, offers the ability to directly assess the contour of the distal radius articular surface.

Studies comparing dorsal to volar plating for distal radius fractures have found similar rates of loss of fixation between the two approaches. In a retrospective cohort comparison of 57 dorsal and 47 volar plate fixations for distal radius fractures, each group had one case of loss of reduction [46]. Similar findings were reported in a comparison study for 29 AO type C3 fractures, in which 14 dorsal and 15 volar plates were used for definitive fixation [47]. Two fractures lost fixation in the dorsal plate group, while only one lost fixation in the volar plate group. In a larger study conducted by Wichlas et al. comparing volar to dorsal locking plates, the authors report the average changes in dorsal tilt and ulnar variance within each group [48]. In this study, 95 % of the 60 dorsal plates were used for AO type C3 fractures, whereas only 56 % of 225 volar plates were used for type C3 fractures. Statistically significant differences were found in measurements of volar tilt and ulnar variance in favor of the volar plating group, however, differences of 2° of dorsal tilt, and 0.6 mm of radial shortening may not be clinically relevant, and the volar plates were, on average, used in less severe fractures.

Management

When considering how to manage loss of fixation in distal radius fractures, the patient's goals regarding function and pain should be clearly established prior to making treatment decision. Radiographic evidence of loss of reduction does not always correlate with poor subjective or clinical outcomes, and it is common for patients to electively forgo further surgical intervention to correct the deformity. Generally speaking, young, active patients with high functional demands deserve restoration of acceptable anatomic relationships to give them the best chance of long-term satisfaction, whereas more elderly patients, many with comorbidities, may be better served with conservative management if their goals do not warrant a more aggressive approach.

Revision surgery typically requires removal of old hardware, correction of the most egregious elements of deformity, and placement of new hardware to reestablish anatomic relationships. These three goals represent the steps in revision surgery of the distal radius, and they also represent the key challenges. In general, our approach is to first determine the most irritating element after fixation failure. If hardware is in the joint, then removal of hardware alone may suffice to improve symptoms. If radial shortening is the cause of symptoms, then patients are typically symptomatic at their less injured ulnar side. If volar dislocation of the carpus has occurred, then the hardware may be a smaller factor than the inadequate fixation. In general, we approach the cause of the patients discomfort as the primary goal for corrective surgery.

One general principle is that revision surgery for loss of fixation may be from a side opposite the previous fixation. Failed volar plates can be stabilized with either temporary or permanent dorsal plates. However this is not an unbreakable rule, and loss of volar fixation due to shearing volar Barton-type injuries may be best addressed with revision volar fixation. Dorsal comminution can also lead to fixation failure. Screws penetrating the joint from the volar side should be removed and temporary fixation, using either a spanning wrist plate or external fixation, may suffice to maintain a newly corrected distal radius position until healing has sufficiently occurred. When percutaneous pinning fails to maintain the position of the distal radius, then volar or dorsal plating can suffice to address the problem. Often supplemental allograft can be employed to provide mechanical support.

A special consideration should be made regarding the timing of surgery. Sometimes it is more appropriate to keep a patient immobilized at the wrist and focus on finger ROM during a convalescent period when fixation is known to be inadequate, simply to maintain or regain finger ROM in preparation for revision surgery. The revision surgery does not necessarily require an early intervention at the wrist, especially if it is being done at the expense of finger ROM. Oftentimes the initial 6-week healing period is lost and reestablishing finger ROM with aggressive therapy and interventions is most beneficial. If loss of fixation is contributing to loss of ROM in the fingers, then early intervention is often more appropriate, as is the case when screws penetrate the cortex from the dorsal side and irritate the tendons. In such cases, rigid fixation, even if temporary, should be maintained at the time of revision surgery with attention paid to the tendons that animate the fingers. This is often the case when percutaneous pinning has failed, but also can be seen in loss of fixation of the critical volar fragment of the radius.

References

1. Beumer A, McQueen MM. Fractures of the distal radius in low-demand elderly patients: closed reduction of no value in 53 of 60 wrists. Acta Orthop Scand. 2003;74:98–100.
2. Egol KA, Walsh M, Romo-Cardoso S, Dorsky S, Paksima N. Distal radial fractures in the elderly: operative compared with nonoperative treatment. J Bone Joint Surg Am. 2010;92:1851–7.
3. Clement ND, Duckworth AD, Court-Brown CM, McQueen MM. Distal radial fractures in the superelderly: does malunion affect functional outcome? ISRN Orthop. 2014;2014:189803.
4. Berglund LM, Messer TM. Complications of volar plate fixation for managing distal radius fractures. J Am Acad Orthop Surg. 2009;17:369–77.
5. Graham TJ. Surgical correction of malunited fractures of the distal radius. J Am Acad Orthop Surg. 1997;5:270–81.
6. Lafontaine M, Hardy D, Delince P. Stability assessment of distal radius fractures. Injury. 1989;20:208–10.
7. Mackenney PJ, McQueen MM, Elton R. Prediction of instability in distal radial fractures. J Bone Joint Surg Am. 2006;88:1944–51.
8. Orbay JL. The treatment of unstable distal radius fractures with volar fixation. Hand Surg. 2000;5:103–12.
9. Orbay JL, Fernandez DL. Volar fixation for dorsally displaced fractures of the distal radius: a preliminary report. J Hand Surg Am. 2002;27:205–15.
10. Drobetz H, Kutscha-Lissberg E. Osteosynthesis of distal radial fractures with a volar locking screw plate system. Int Orthop. 2003;27:1–6.
11. Drobetz H, Bryant AL, Pokorny T, Spitaler R, Leixnering M, Jupiter JB. Volar fixed-angle plating of distal radius extension fractures: influence of plate position on secondary loss of reduction–a biomechanic study in a cadaveric model. J Hand Surg Am. 2006;31:615–22.

12. Nygaard M, Nielsen NS, Bojsen-Moller F. A biomechanical evaluation of the relative load change in the joints of the wrist with ulnar shortening: a 'handbag' model. J Hand Surg Eur Vol. 2009;34:724–9.

13. Palmer AK, Werner FW. Biomechanics of the distal radioulnar joint. Clin Orthop Relat Res. 1984;26–35.

14. Tencer AF, Viegas SF, Cantrell J, Chang M, Clegg P, Hicks C, O'Meara C, Williamson JB. Pressure distribution in the wrist joint. J Orthop Res. 1988;6:509–17.

15. Bronstein AJ, Trumble TE, Tencer AF. The effects of distal radius fracture malalignment on forearm rotation: a cadaveric study. J Hand Surg Am. 1997;22:258–62.

16. Beumer A, Adlercreutz C, Lindau TR. Early prognostic factors in distal radius fractures in a younger than osteoporotic age group: a multivariate analysis of trauma radiographs. BMC Musculoskelet Disord. 2013;14:170.

17. Short WH, Palmer AK, Werner FW, Murphy DJ. A biomechanical study of distal radial fractures. J Hand Surg Am. 1987;12:529–34.

18. Leung F, Ozkan M, Chow SP. Conservative treatment of intra-articular fractures of the distal radius–factors affecting functional outcome. Hand Surg. 2000;5:145–53.

19. Wilcke MK, Abbaszadegan H, Adolphson PY. Patient-perceived outcome after displaced distal radius fractures. A comparison between radiological parameters, objective physical variables, and the DASH score. J Hand Ther. 2007;20:290–8. quiz 299.

20. Pogue DJ, Viegas SF, Patterson RM, Peterson PD, Jenkins DK, Sweo TD, Hokanson JA. Effects of distal radius fracture malunion on wrist joint mechanics. J Hand Surg Am. 1990;15:721–7.

21. Karnezis IA, Panagiotopoulos E, Tyllianakis M, Megas P, Lambiris E. Correlation between radiological parameters and patient-rated wrist dysfunction following fractures of the distal radius. Injury. 2005; 36:1435–9.

22. McQueen M, Caspers J. Colles fracture: does the anatomical result affect the final function? J Bone Joint Surg Br. 1988;70:649–51.

23. Jupiter JB. Fractures of the distal end of the radius. J Bone Joint Surg Am. 1991;73:461–9.

24. Hudak PL, Amadio PC, Bombardier C. Development of an upper extremity outcome measure: the DASH (disabilities of the arm, shoulder and hand) [corrected]. The Upper Extremity Collaborative Group (UECG). Am J Ind Med. 1996;29:602–8.

25. Brogren E, Hofer M, Petranek M, Wagner P, Dahlin LB, Atroshi I. Relationship between distal radius fracture malunion and arm-related disability: a prospective population-based cohort study with 1-year follow-up. BMC Musculoskelet Disord. 2011;12:9.

26. Lundy DW, Quisling SG, Lourie GM, Feiner CM, Lins RE. Tilted lateral radiographs in the evaluation of intra-articular distal radius fractures. J Hand Surg Am. 1999;24:249–56.

27. Andermahr J, Lozano-Calderon S, Trafton T, Crisco JJ, Ring D. The volar extension of the lunate facet of the distal radius: a quantitative anatomic study. J Hand Surg Am. 2006;31:892–5.
28. Beck JD, Harness NG, Spencer HT. Volar plate fixation failure for volar shearing distal radius fractures with small lunate facet fragments. J Hand Surg Am. 2014;39:670–8.
29. Glickel SZ, Catalano LW, Raia FJ, Barron OA, Grabow R, Chia B. Long-term outcomes of closed reduction and percutaneous pinning for the treatment of distal radius fractures. J Hand Surg Am. 2008;33:1700–5.
30. Clancey GJ. Percutaneous Kirschner-wire fixation of Colles fractures. A prospective study of thirty cases. J Bone Joint Surg Am. 1984;66: 1008–14.
31. Mah ET, Atkinson RN. Percutaneous Kirschner wire stabilisation following closed reduction of Colles' fractures. J Hand Surg Br. 1992; 17:55–62.
32. Botte MJ, Davis JL, Rose BA, von Schroeder HP, Gellman H, Zinberg EM, Abrams RA. Complications of smooth pin fixation of fractures and dislocations in the hand and wrist. Clin Orthop Relat Res. 1992;(276):194–201.
33. Rosati M, Bertagnini S, Digrandi G, Sala C. Percutaneous pinning for fractures of the distal radius. Acta Orthop Belg. 2006;72:138–46.
34. Yang TY, Tsai YH, Shen SH, Huang KC. Radiographic outcomes of percutaneous pinning for displaced extra-articular fractures of the distal radius: a time course study. Biomed Res Int. 2014;2014:540874.
35. Barton T, Chambers C, Lane E, Bannister G. Do Kirschner wires maintain reduction of displaced Colles' fractures? Injury. 2005;36:1431–4.
36. Rizzo M, Katt BA, Carothers JT. Comparison of locked volar plating versus pinning and external fixation in the treatment of unstable intraarticular distal radius fractures. Hand (N Y). 2008;3:111–7.
37. Kennedy C, Kennedy MT, Niall D, Devitt A. Radiological outcomes of distal radius extra-articular fragility fractures treated with extra-focal Kirschner wires. Injury. 2010;41:639–42.
38. Kim JY, Tae SK. Percutaneous distal radius-ulna pinning of distal radius fractures to prevent settling. J Hand Surg Am. 2014;39:1921–5.
39. Rozental TD, Blazar PE. Functional outcome and complications after volar plating for dorsally displaced, unstable fractures of the distal radius. J Hand Surg Am. 2006;31:359–65.
40. Gogna P, Selhi HS, Singla R, Devgan A, Magu NK, Mahindra P, Yamin M. Dorsally comminuted fractures of the distal end of the radius: osteosynthesis with volar fixed angle locking plates. ISRN Orthop. 2013; 2013:131757.
41. Arora R, Lutz M, Hennerbichler A, Krappinger D, Espen D, Gabl M. Complications following internal fixation of unstable distal radius fracture with a palmar locking-plate. J Orthop Trauma. 2007;21:316–22.
42. Harness NG, Jupiter JB, Orbay JL, Raskin KB, Fernandez DL. Loss of fixation of the volar lunate facet fragment in fractures of the distal part of the radius. J Bone Joint Surg Am. 2004;86-A:1900–8.

43. Kamath AF, Zurakowski D, Day CS. Low-profile dorsal plating for dorsally angulated distal radius fractures: an outcomes study. J Hand Surg Am. 2006;31:1061–7.
44. Simic PM, Robison J, Gardner MJ, Gelberman RH, Weiland AJ, Boyer MI. Treatment of distal radius fractures with a low-profile dorsal plating system: an outcomes assessment. J Hand Surg Am. 2006;31:382–6.
45. Ruch DS, Papadonikolakis A. Volar versus dorsal plating in the management of intra-articular distal radius fractures. J Hand Surg Am. 2006;31:9–16.
46. Yu YR, Makhni MC, Tabrizi S, Rozental TD, Mundanthanam G, Day CS. Complications of low-profile dorsal versus volar locking plates in the distal radius: a comparative study. J Hand Surg Am. 2011;36:1135–41.
47. Rein S, Schikore H, Schneiders W, Amlang M, Zwipp H. Results of dorsal or volar plate fixation of AO type C3 distal radius fractures: a retrospective study. J Hand Surg Am. 2007;32:954–61.
48. Wichlas F, Haas NP, Disch A, Macho D, Tsitsilonis S. Complication rates and reduction potential of palmar versus dorsal locking plate osteosynthesis for the treatment of distal radius fractures. J Orthop Traumatol. 2014;15:259–64.

Chapter 18
Distal Radius Fracture Complicated by Carpal Tunnel Syndrome

Caroline N. Wolfe, Nikhil R. Oak and Jeffrey N. Lawton

Case Presentation

A 72-year-old right-hand-dominant woman presented to the emergency department after a ground-level fall with pain in her right wrist and limited wrist motion due to pain (Fig. 18.1). She had no complaints of numbness or tingling. She was placed in a sugar-tong splint and transitioned to a well-molded cast in fingertraps at 1 week. She presented to clinic at 2 weeks with a substantial increase of dorsal tilt but declined surgery (Fig. 18.2). At 3 weeks, she had more loss of dorsal tilt and described progressive numbness in the thumb, index, and middle fingers (Fig. 18.3). Based upon her worsening deformity and median nerve dysfunction, she was then taken to the operating room and underwent open reduction and internal fixation of her right distal radius fracture (DRF) and median nerve decompression. Postoperative radiographs showed restoration of distal radius palmar tilt (Fig. 18.4). She also regained full wrist range of motion and sensation in the median nerve distribution postoperatively (Fig. 18.5).

C.N. Wolfe • N.R. Oak • J.N. Lawton, MD (✉)
Department of Orthopaedic Surgery, University of Michigan Health System, A. Alfred Taubman Health Care Center, Floor 2, Reception: B, 2912 Taubman Center, 1500 East Medical Center Drive, Ann Arbor, MI 48109-5328, USA
e-mail: jeflawto@med.umich.edu

© Springer International Publishing Switzerland 2016
J.N. Lawton (ed.), *Distal Radius Fractures*,
DOI 10.1007/978-3-319-27489-8_18

229

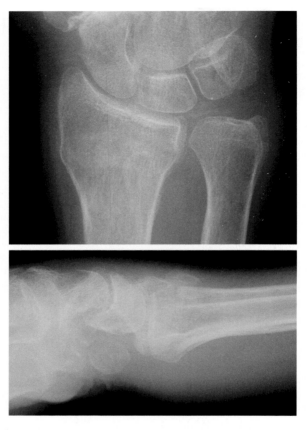

Fig. 18.1 Initial posteroanterior (*top*) and lateral (*bottom*) radiographs demonstrate a minimally impacted right distal radius fracture with neutral palmar tilt

Background

DRFs are the most common type of fracture seen in the emergency department. Reported incidence is 640,000 per year in the USA [1]. Several complications may occur with treatment of a DRF, including persistent neuropathy, radiocarpal or radioulnar arthrosis, malunion, nonunion, tendon rupture, complex regional pain syndrome,

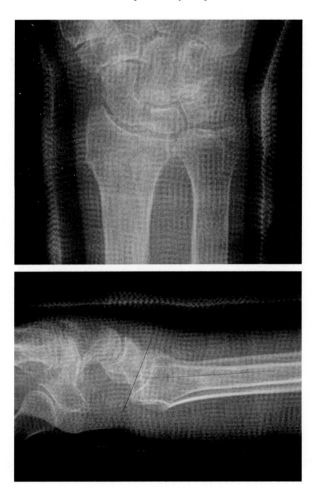

Fig. 18.2 At 2-week follow-up, patient demonstrated loss of palmar tilt on the lateral radiograph (*bottom*). Palmar tilt is measured by an angle between a line along the distal radial articular surface and a line perpendicular to the longitudinal axis of the radius. When this angle is 90°, palmar tilt is zero. Palmar tilt is identified with a plus sign and dorsal tilt with a minus sign. Normal tilt averages +11 but can range from −7 to +28 [17]. This patient shows dorsal tilt of approximately −20 (*bottom*)

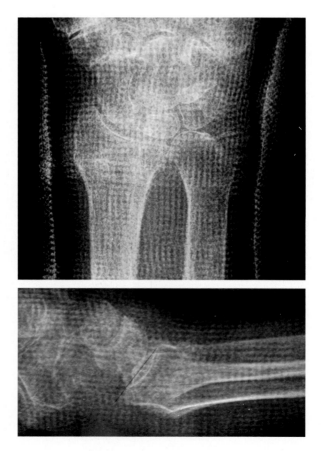

Fig. 18.3 After 1 additional week, repeat lateral radiograph showing further loss of palmar tilt to approximately −30 (*bottom*)

ulnar impaction, loss of forearm rotation, digital stiffness and, rarely, compartment syndrome [1, 2]. Carpal tunnel syndrome (CTS) is a well-described complication following DRF, with a reported incidence of 3.3 % to 17.2 % [3, 4]. CTS can develop early, or several months to years following DRF. Several studies have investigated the causes of CTS after DRF and discussed the

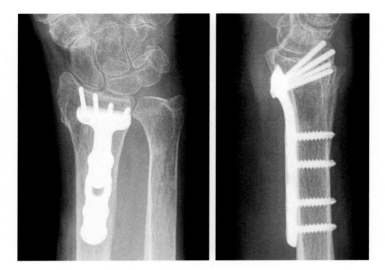

Fig. 18.4 Postoperative posteroanterior (*left*) and lateral (*right*) radiographs showing stable volar plate fixation of the distal radius fracture and restoration of palmar tilt (*right*)

predisposing risk factures. Failure to recognize acute symptoms of median nerve compression can lead to a delay in treatment and permanent nerve dysfunction or pain following a DRF.

Anatomy

In 1854 Sir James Paget [5] first described symptoms of CTS after DRFs when excessive callus formation compressed the median nerve [3, 6]. The dorsal border of the carpal tunnel is composed of the concave arch of the carpus. Volarly, the transverse carpal ligament encloses the carpal tunnel. The anteroposterior depth of the carpal tunnel measures from 10 to 13 mm at its deepest point. Ten structures pass through the carpal tunnel, including nine flexor tendons and the median nerve. The median nerve is the most superficial component, passing through the space just radial to midline,

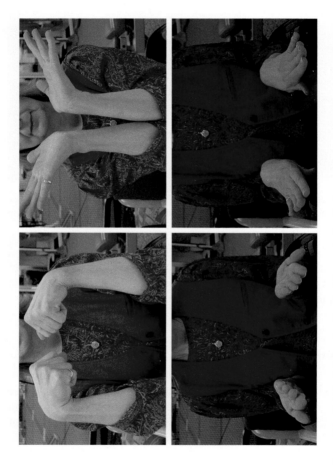

Fig. 18.5 Postoperative clinical photographs of patient demonstrating flexion, extension, supination, and pronation

and is covered by a layer of cellulo-adipose tissue [7, 8]. Vance and Gelberman [9] demonstrated that the distance of the median nerve to the radius is approximately 3 mm at the level of the wrist.

As pressure within the carpal tunnel increases, perfusion to the epineurium of the median nerve decreases, which causes ischemia. This can lead to a block in nerve conduction and dysfunction in axonal transport, and it may symptomatically present as numbness and paraesthesia [10]. Untreated CTS following a DRF can lead to permanent dysfunction of the median nerve and an increased risk for the development of chronic regional pain syndrome.

Diagnosis

Patients often report numbness, pain, or burning within the median nerve distribution that can include all or part of the thumb, index, and middle fingers as well as the radial half of the ring finger. Chronic CTS can cause weakness with thumb opposition as well as thenar muscle atrophy [8]. Specific tests to diagnosis CTS include Phalen's test, increased symptoms with prolonged wrist flexion, or Tinel's test, percussion over the median nerve at the wrist and palm. Durkan's test, direct compression of the median nerve at the carpal tunnel, has a sensitivity of 87 % and a specificity of 90 % in detecting CTS [8]. However, direct compression may be difficult in the setting of acute fracture. Testing for median nerve sensation and palpation for thenar muscular contraction upon attempted palmar abduction and opposition should be done in the setting of an acute DRF to ensure nerve function. A change in two-point discrimination over time is useful in diagnosing and distinguishing acute CTS from immediate nerve contusion.

Carpal Tunnel Syndrome

The onset of CTS after a DRF ranges from several hours to years. It can be divided into acute or early, and delayed or late, which can occur months to years after injury. Late CTS is a form of chronic

CTS and is associated with malunion, chronic edema, prolonged immobilization in wrist flexion, or excessive callus formation [1, 8]. In 1980, Cooney and colleagues [11] reviewed 565 patients with Colles' fractures and reported compression neuropathy to be the most frequent single complication at 7.9 %. Early median neuropathy developed in 31 patients. Late neuropathy of the median nerve occurred in 45 patients and 31 of these patients required release of the carpal tunnel [11]. Stewart et al. [12] found that CTS developed acutely and chronically after DRF and reported 17 % development of CTS at 3 months after injury and another 12 % at 6 months after injury in 100 patients with DRFs.

Risk factors for developing CTS are multifactorial. Idiopathic is the most common etiology, with the patient experiencing progressive median nerve paresthesia that worsens with repetitive activity or wrist flexion. CTS can also occur with anatomic changes in the carpal tunnel after DRF and chronic inflammation or edema of the tenosynovium. Delayed CTS after DRF has been reported to range from 0.5 % to 22 % [1, 8].

Acute CTS after DRF has a reported occurrence of 5.4 % to 8.6 % [1]. It develops slowly over hours to days after initial injury and occurs due to a rapid increase in pressure within the carpal tunnel, causing progressive paresthesias. Immediately at the time of injury it must be distinguished from median nerve dysfunction arising from nerve contusion or neuropraxia by volar displaced fracture fragments. Patients with nerve contusion or neuropraxia present with initial paresthesia that often improves with fracture reduction. Acute CTS most likely requires immediate surgical decompression to prevent permanent nerve dysfunction [13].

Pathomechanics

Since CTS can occur at various time periods following a DRF, there are multiple reported mechanisms for development. One major cause of acute CTS is acute changes in canal pressures. Hematoma formation from trauma to the distal radius can extravasate into the carpal tunnel, increasing canal pressures. The degree of trauma relates with magnitude of hemorrhage [4, 14]. Kongsholm and Olerud [14] found higher canal pressures with increasing severity of fracture. With higher fracture severity there seems to be greater tissue damage that leads to more bleeding and edema, increasing pressure within the carpal tunnel. Itsubo et al. [4] reviewed 105 wrists with CTS following DRF and reported that 68 % of the acute onset group had a multifragmented and intra-articular type fracture, and 46 % were associated with high-energy trauma. In the subacute (1–12 weeks) and delayed onset group (12+ weeks), 79 % and 63 %, respectively, had A-type fractures and more than 90 % were associated with low-energy trauma [4].

Kongsholm and Olerud [14] also described two additional factors that contribute to an increase in pressure within the carpal tunnel in the acute stage of Colles' fracture. Carpal canal pressures can increase with injection of local anesthetic into the fracture hematoma at the time of reduction [14]. Also, placement of the wrist in the Cotton-Loder position, which involves dramatic wrist flexion and ulnar deviation, significantly increases carpal tunnel pressure and the risk of median compression [3]. Kongsholm and Olerud [14] found that for every degree of increased volar flexion, carpal tunnel pressure increased 0.8 mm Hg [14]. Gelberman et al. [15] found that intracarpal canal interstitial fluid pressures increased from 18 mm Hg in neutral wrist position to 47 mm Hg in 40° of flexion in wrists with Colles' fractures.

Paget [5] described CTS following DRFs and related the complication to excessive volar callus formation [3, 6]. Cooney et al. [11], in 1980, reported that chronic CTS was related to volar fracture fragments, excessive callus formation, persistent hematoma, and localized swelling. Excessive callus formation or malunion causes narrowing of the cross-sectional area of the carpal tunnel [3, 16]. In 1984, Taleisnik and Watson [17] found that the loss of the normal palmar tilt of the distal articular surface of the radius predisposes the patient to midcarpal instability. This involves dorsal angulation of the lunate and flexion of the midcarpal joint, thereby narrowing the carpal tunnel [17]. In 1988, Aro et al. [16] reviewed 166 Colles' fractures treated conservatively and reported an 8 % rate of late median nerve compression neuropathy, diagnosed at follow-up exam. Eighty-five percent of patients with median nerve compression had a malunion with radial collapse or dorsal angulation, causing narrowing of the carpal tunnel [16].

In 1963, Lynch and Lipscomb [3] described nonspecific tenosynovitis, inflammation of the flexor tendon synovitis, following DRF to increase the volume of the structures within the carpal tunnel, leading to median nerve compression.

Treatment

According to the adult DRF treatment guidelines of 2009 [18], the American Academy of Orthopaedic Surgeons (AAOS) was unable to recommend for or against performing nerve decompression when nerve dysfunction persists after reduction of DRF due to inconclusive evidence. Patients may have spontaneous resolution of symptoms after DRF fixation [1, 18].

In a retrospective case–control study, Dyer et al. [13] reported that fracture translation was the most important risk factor for acute CTS in patients who underwent open reduction and internal fixation of a DRF. They recommended prophylactic carpal tunnel release (CTR) in female patients younger than 48 years with 35 % fracture translation [13].

However, Odumala et al. [19] evaluated prophylactic carpal tunnel decompression and its effects on median nerve dysfunction after DRF fixation. An extended incision to the ulnar side of the thenar eminence was performed in a group of patients who underwent carpal tunnel decompression. The authors found that patients who had prophylactic carpal tunnel decompression at the time of DRF fixation were twice as likely to have acute median nerve dysfunction, which may increase postoperative morbidity [19]. Several studies have considered release of the carpal tunnel endoscopically or through a separate incision. Weber and Sanders [20] described the flexor carpi radialis (FCR) approach to carpal tunnel decompression and its benefits, including direct visualization of the carpal tunnel and decreased disruption of skin and soft tissues directly over the median nerve. Gwathmey et al. [21] studied prophylactic carpal tunnel decompression at the time of volar plate osteosynthesis using a hybrid FCR approach with a radial-sided release of the transverse carpal ligament and found decreased signs or symptoms of acute CTS. [21] Therefore, if concomitant CTR is required at the time of distal radius fixation, it may be performed through a separate incision or through a hybrid FCR approach [1]. Median nerve symptoms associated with DRF, however, may be due to stretch/direct contusion to the median nerve itself, instead of secondary to compression as is seen in CTS. As such, CTR may improve the environment and allow for quicker improvement of symptoms, but patients must be warned that CTR may not result in prompt or immediate relief of symptoms.

Conclusion

CTS is a well-described complication following DRFs. Onset of symptoms can vary from hours to years after injury. It is important to identify the risks of median nerve compression such as local anesthetic hematoma-block injection, immobilization in a Cotton-Loder position, or malunion. Delayed CTS can be treated similar to chronic carpal tunnel in the general population. Although prophylactic CTR at the time of distal radius fixation has not been recommended by the AAOS, it is important to recognize and treat acute CTS when symptoms occur. Lack of early recognition can lead to a delay in diagnosis and treatment, which can cause permanent nerve dysfunction.

References

1. Niver GE, Ilyas AM. Carpal tunnel syndrome after distal radius fracture. Orthop Clin North Am. 2012;43(4):521–7.
2. Wolfe S. Green's operative hand surgery. 6th ed. Philadelphia: Elsevier/Churchill Livingstone; 2010.
3. Lynch AC, Lipscomb PR. The carpal tunnel syndrome and Colles' fractures. JAMA. 1963;185:363–6.
4. Itsubo T, Hayashi M, Uchiyama S, Hirachi K, Minami A, Kato H. Differential onset patterns and causes of carpal tunnel syndrome after distal radius fracture: a retrospective study of 105 wrists. J Orthop Sci. 2010;15(4):518–23.

5. Paget J. Lectures on surgical pathology. Philadelphia: Lindsay & Blakiston; 1854. p. 42.
6. Paley D, McMurtry RY. Median nerve compression by volarly displaced fragments of the distal radius. Clin Orthop Relat Res. 1987;215:139–47.
7. Rotman MB, Donovan JP. Practical anatomy of the carpal tunnel. Hand Clin. 2002;18(2):219–30.
8. Cranford CS, Ho JY, Kalainov DM, Hartigan BJ. Carpal tunnel syndrome. J Am Acad Orthop Surg. 2007;15(9):537–48.
9. Vance RM, Gelberman RH. Acute ulnar neuropathy with fractures at the wrist. J Bone Joint Surg Am. 1978;60(7):962–5.
10. Tosti R, Ilyas AM. Acute carpal tunnel syndrome. Orthop Clin North Am. 2012;43(4):459–65.
11. Cooney 3rd WP, Dobyns JH, Linscheid RL. Complications of Colles' fractures. J Bone Joint Surg Am. 1980;62(4):613–9.
12. Stewart HD, Innes AR, Burke FD. The hand complications of Colles' fractures. J Hand Surg Br. 1985;10(1):103–6.
13. Dyer G, Lozano-Calderon S, Gannon C, Baratz M, Ring D. Predictors of acute carpal tunnel syndrome associated with fracture of the distal radius. J Hand Surg Am. 2008;33(8):1309–13.
14. Kongsholm J, Olerud C. Carpal tunnel pressure in the acute phase after Colles' fracture. Arch Orthop Trauma Surg. 1986;105(3):183–6.
15. Gelberman RH, Szabo RM, Mortensen WW. Carpal tunnel pressures and wrist position in patients with Colles' fractures. J Trauma. 1984;24(8): 747–9.
16. Aro H, Koivunen T, Katevuo K, Nieminen S, Aho AJ. Late compression neuropathies after Colles' fractures. Clin Orthop Relat Res. 1988;233: 217–25.
17. Taleisnik J, Watson HK. Midcarpal instability caused by malunited fractures of the distal radius. J Hand Surg Am. 1984;9(3):350–7.
18. Lichtman DM, Bindra RR, Boyer MI, et al. Treatment of distal radius fractures. J Am Acad Orthop Surg. 2010;18(3):180–9.
19. Odumala O, Ayekoloye C, Packer G. Prophylactic carpal tunnel decompression during buttress plating of the distal radius–is it justified? Injury. 2001;32(7):577–9.
20. Weber RA, Sanders WE. Flexor carpi radialis approach for carpal tunnel release. J Hand Surg Am. 1997;22(1):120–6.
21. Gwathmey Jr FW, Brunton LM, Pensy RA, Chhabra AB. Volar plate osteosynthesis of distal radius fractures with concurrent prophylactic carpal tunnel release using a hybrid flexor carpi radialis approach. J Hand Surg Am. 2010;35(7):1082–8. e1084.

Chapter 19
Complications of Distal Radius Fracture: EPL Rupture

Benjamin L. Gray and Andrew D. Markiewitz

A Case Series

Patient 1

A 54-year-old right hand dominant woman was involved in a motor vehicle accident. She was evaluated with a closed reduction performed in the Emergency Department. After leaving the Emergency Department, she noted significant numbness and tingling in the thumb and index finger reporting it upon presentation to the Hand Surgeon. Given the significant dorsal comminution as well as the median nerve symptoms, operative fixation and a carpal tunnel release were undertaken within the week. One month later, she felt a painful pop on the dorsum of her wrist and was unable to

B.L. Gray, MD (✉)
Department of Orthopaedic Surgery, University of Pennsylvania Health System, Pennsylvania Hospital, 800 Spruce St, 1 Cathcart Building, Philadelphia, PA 19107, USA
e-mail: Benjamin.Gray@uphs.upenn.edu

A.D. Markiewitz, MD
Department of Orthopaedic Surgery, Trihealth Inc., 16500 Montgomery Rd, 150, Cincinnati, OH 45234, USA
e-mail: dettdoc@ad.com

© Springer International Publishing Switzerland 2016   241
J.N. Lawton (ed.), *Distal Radius Fractures*,
DOI 10.1007/978-3-319-27489-8_19

extend her thumb at the interphalangeal joint. No prominent screws were visualized at the time of surgery in the third or fourth compartments (Fig. 19.1).

Patient 2

A 54-year-old woman fell while roller skating and fractured her distal radius. She was initially splinted and transitioned to a cast for a nondisplaced distal radius fracture. She noted 4 weeks after the injury that she could flex her thumb but not extend it. At the time of surgery, she was found to have ruptured her EPL. Radiographs throughout her clinical course demonstrated her continued nondisplaced fracture.

Patient 3

A 38-year-old woman fell from a bar stool onto her right arm. She fractured her distal radius and was initially treated nonoperatively with a splint followed by a brace at 2 weeks. The patient noted increased pain and tightness around her thumb. Her fracture had displaced. She thus underwent ORIF of her distal radius 4 weeks after the injury. Four weeks after surgery, she noted inability to extend her thumb. Screws were noted to be prominent in the area of the metaphyseal distal radius (Fig. 19.2). The plate was removed and the transfer was performed dorsally to restore function to her thumb.

Based upon clinical examination, the diagnosis in each case was a rupture of the extensor pollicis longus tendon at the level of Lister's tubercle. These three cases represent three different faces of the same complication. The EPL remnant, distally, allowed transfer of the extensor indicis proprius with transfer to the first metacarpal level in all three cases.

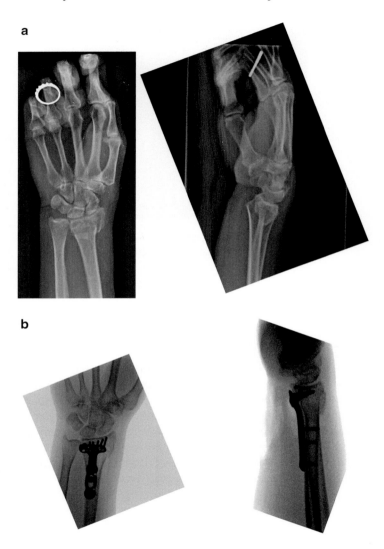

Fig. 19.1 Spontaneous rupture. (**a**) Initial radiographs at the time of injury demonstrate a comminuted dorsally displaced distal radius fracture. (**b**) Postoperative fluoroscopy films demonstrate an adequate reduction with screws that are not prominent dorsally

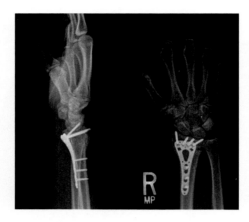

Fig. 19.2 Prominent screws dorsally. Postoperative radiographs taken at the time of follow-up demonstrate an adequate reduction but prominent screws dorsally

Etiology

Rupture of the extensor pollicis longus tendon is a well-known complication of distal radius fractures. It occurs in 0.07–5 % of nondisplaced fractures treated nonoperatively and up to 2–8.6 % of those treated operatively with a volar plate [1–4]. The rupture commonly occurs between 1 and 3 months after the injury with the characteristic inability to extend the thumb. There are various theories as to the etiology of the rupture and thus we break our selection into two separate categories: nondisplaced fractures treated in a cast and dorsally displaced fractures treated with a volar plate.

For the nondisplaced fracture, there are multiple factors proposed. Previous studies have demonstrated the poor vascularity of the extensor pollicis longus at the level of Lister's tubercle. This is a watershed area of the tendon as there are separate proximal and distal intrinsic vascular systems [5]. In a nondisplaced fracture, there is not enough force to rupture the extensor retinaculum. Thus it is maintained as a constrictive environment.

As a hematoma develops from the fracture, the pressure builds up within the fibro-osseous tunnel of the third dorsal compartment. This decreases the synovial production and can jeopardize the vascularity to the tendon. Other factors can also decrease the space within the canal such as sharp, bony ossicles extending up from the fracture or callous formation that develops as the fracture heals.

With displaced fractures, the sheath may rupture allowing the tendon to displace out of its tight tract. Thus, there may be three forms of iatrogenic injuries to the tendon. If the fracture is close reduced, there is the possibility that the tendon can become entrapped within the fracture and possibly injured. In placing the distal locking screws for a volar distal radius plate, the drill has been reported to penetrate too deeply and injure the tendon dorsally [4]. The final possibility is that screw can be placed too long, leaving a prominent screw within the groove of the third or fourth dorsal compartment that leads to a repetitive abrasion of the tendon with ultimate rupture [6].

Diagnosis

The diagnosis can most often be made clinically. Patients will present with the complaint that they can flex but no longer extend their thumb. Advanced diagnostic testing is not usually needed. Occasionally, they will feel a pop or describe pain dorsally over their wrist prior to the event. In some situations, a prodrome of dorsal wrist pain with thumb motion that develops after the patient's fracture pain seems to subside can lead to a diagnosis of tendinitis of the extensor. Early transposition may prevent rupture of the tendon. Once the tendon has ruptured, the attrition damage prevents primary repair.

If clinical acumen is insufficient, one may order an ultrasound to confirm the diagnosis. With ultrasound, a tubular hypoechoic area replaces the normal tendon which corresponds to a fluid-filled or hemorrhagic synovial sheath [7]. Ultrasound better defines the amount of retraction of the tendon as well.

Prevention

There are several ways to decrease the risk of extensor pollicis longus tendon injury in the operating room. Fluoroscopic assessment of screw length during surgery can minimize this risk by using special views. With the standard lateral film of the distal radius, a prominent screw within the third compartment can be shrouded by Lister's tubercle. Thus, the screw length may appear appropriate when in reality it has penetrated the cortex dorsally. Ozer et al. found that the lateral view was 68 % sensitive for screw penetration of 1 mm and 80 % sensitive for screws that penetrated 2 mm [8]. They advocated for a dorsal tangential view to better assess if a screw was prominent. In this view, the wrist is flexed, and the beam is placed tangential to the dorsal surface to better define screw penetration (Fig. 19.3).

The other technique utilized is to adjust the screw length. Classic teaching was that bicortical fixation was the standard for all distal radius fractures. Wall et al. studied the effect of screw length on stability and found that unicortical screws representing 75 % of the bone width (75 % of the measured depth) had similar stiffness to bicortical fixation [9].

Thus with locking plate fixation, screws can be shortened to protect the extensor tendons.

Treatment

Typically a primary repair of the EPL is not possible given the attrition damage and atrophic nature of the tendon. Our standard treatment for rupture of the extensor pollicis longus tendon is to perform a transfer of the extensor indicis proprius tendon to the extensor pollicis longus remnant distally. These muscles have similar excursion and direction of pull. This transfer can be performed through three small incisions (Fig. 19.4a). The first incision is made proximal to the thumb MCP joint and the EPL is identified. The tendon remnant can be explored first to determine if a longer slip of the EIP is necessary. One should be cautious in this area as a branch of the

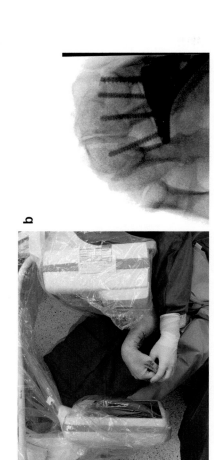

Fig. 19.3 Dorsal tangential view of the radius. (**a**) Proper positioning for the radiograph is important with the wrist flexed. (**b**) This view provides an excellent view of the dorsal cortex and is sensitive for screw penetration. Notice that no screws are prominent

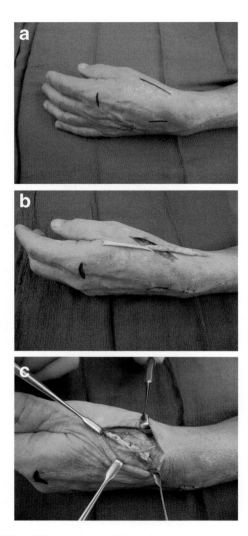

Fig. 19.4 EIP to EPL transfer. (**a**) Three separate incisions are marked out. The first is proximal to the thumb MCP joint and is longitudinal where the Pulvertaft weave will take place. The second is just proximal to the MCP joint of the index finger. The last is at the level of the wrist just ulnar to Lister's tubercle. (**b**) The extensor indicis proprius has been transected at the level of the MCP joint and tunneled from the proximal wound at the wrist to the thumb. The EIP lays distally and the ruptured end of the EPL lays proximal. (**c**) The Pulvertaft weave is evident in the wound. Note that the tendon transfer is performed deep to the branch of the superficial radial nerve

superficial radial nerve can be present. The transfer should be made below this nerve branch. Injury to the nerve or placing the transfer above it can lead to postoperative neuralgia and chronic pain. The second incision is made proximal to the index finger metacarpophalangeal joint. The EIP is identified as the ulnar tendon to the EDCindex. Leaving it intact until identified at the wrist does help during the harvest. A third incision is made at the level of the wrist distal to the retinaculum allowing identification of the EIP before transection. The tendon is transected proximal to the sagittal bands and retrieved at the wrist proximally. Occasionally, one does note interconnections between the EDCindex and the EIP which must be lysed to allow for proximal delivery of the tendon. The harvest site could be extended past the sagittal bands and joint if a longer transfer is needed but the gap will need to be repaired. The EIP is then tunneled distally to the EPL remnant subcutaneously (Fig. 19.4b) and a Pulvertaft weave is performed (Fig. 19.4c). If possible, three or four tendon weaves should be performed. The tendon is tensioned with the wrist in neutral and the thumb in full extension. This enables the thumb to flex when the wrist is brought into extension. One should err on the side of a tight repair as a loose repair stays loose with complaints of loss of thumb extension. With the onset of wide awake surgery, some advocate for intraoperative tensioning with the patient awake to aid in appropriate tensioning and to facilitate the reprogramming of the cerebral cortex [10]. Rehabilitation protocols have varied from the traditional immobilization for 3–6 weeks to the early active motion and early dynamic motion protocols [11, 12]. Patients may have decreased independent index finger extension following transfer [13]. We have not seen this problem in our practice; however, high level performers, like pianists, should be warned of this risk. Most patients are quite functional within 8 weeks of transfer.

References

1. Cooney WP, Dobyns JH, Linscheid RL. Complications of Colles' fractures. J Bone Joint Surg Am. 1980;62(4):613–9. http://jbjs.org.beckerproxy. wustl.edu/content/62/4/613.abstract. Accessed 28 Jan 2015.

2. Roth KM, Blazar PE, Earp BE, Han R, Leung A. Incidence of extensor pollicis longus tendon rupture after nondisplaced distal radius fractures. J Hand Surg Am. 2012;37(5):942–7. doi:10.1016/j.jhsa.2012.02.006.

3. Arora R, Lutz M, Hennerbichler A, Krappinger D, Espen D, Gabl M. Complications following internal fixation of unstable distal radius fracture with a palmar locking-plate. J Orthop Trauma. 2007;21(5):316–22. doi:10.1097/BOT.0b013e318059b993.

4. Al-Rashid M, Theivendran K, Craigen MAC. Delayed ruptures of the extensor tendon secondary to the use of volar locking compression plates for distal radial fractures. J Bone Joint Surg Br. 2006;88(12):1610–2. doi:10.1302/0301-620X.88B12.17696.

5. Engkvist O, Lundborg G. Rupture of the extensor pollicis longus tendon after fracture of the lower end of the radius—a clinical and microangiographic study. Hand. 1979;11(1):76–86. http://www.ncbi.nlm.nih.gov/pubmed/488782. Accessed 1 Feb. 2015.

6. Benson EC, DeCarvalho A, Mikola EA, Veitch JM, Moneim MS. Two potential causes of EPL rupture after distal radius volar plate fixation. Clin Orthop Relat Res. 2006;451:218–22. doi:10.1097/01.blo.0000223998.02765.0d.

7. De Maeseneer M, Marcelis S, Osteaux M, Jager T, Machiels F, Van Roy P. Sonography of a rupture of the tendon of the extensor pollicis longus muscle: initial clinical experience and correlation with findings at cadaveric dissection. AJR Am J Roentgenol. 2005;184(1):175–9. doi:10.2214/ajr.184.1.01840175.

8. Ozer K, Wolf JM, Watkins B, Hak DJ. Comparison of 4 fluoroscopic views for dorsal cortex screw penetration after volar plating of the distal radius. J Hand Surg Am. 2012;37(5):963–7. doi:10.1016/j.jhsa.2012.02.026.

9. Wall LB, Brodt MD, Silva MJ, Boyer MI, Calfee RP. The effects of screw length on stability of simulated osteoporotic distal radius fractures fixed with volar locking plates. J Hand Surg Am. 2012;37(3):446–53. doi:10.1016/j.jhsa.2011.12.013.

10. Lalonde DH. Wide-awake extensor indicis proprius to extensor pollicis longus tendon transfer. J Hand Surg Am. 2014;39(11):2297–9. doi:10.1016/j.jhsa.2014.08.024.

11. Germann G, Wagner H, Blome-Eberwein S, Karle B, Wittemann M. Early dynamic motion versus postoperative immobilization in patients with extensor indicis proprius transfer to restore thumb extension: a prospective randomized study. J Hand Surg Am. 2001;26(6):1111–5. doi:10.1053/jhsu.2001.28941.

12. Giessler GA, Przybilski M, Germann G, Sauerbier M, Megerle K. Early free active versus dynamic extension splinting after extensor indicis proprius tendon transfer to restore thumb extension: a prospective randomized study. J Hand Surg Am. 2008;33(6):864–8. doi:10.1016/j.jhsa.2008.01.028.

13. Moore JR, Weiland AJ, Valdata L. Independent index extension after extensor indicis proprius transfer. J Hand Surg Am. 1987;12(2):232–6. doi:10.1016/S0363-5023(87)80277-0.

Index

© Springer International Publishing Switzerland 2016
J.N. Lawton (ed.), *Distal Radius Fractures*,
DOI 10.1007/978-3-319-27489-8

Printed in the United States
By Bookmasters